Success in Academic Surgery

Carla M. Pugh • Rebecca S. Sippel

Editors

Success in Academic Surgery: Developing a Career in Surgical Education

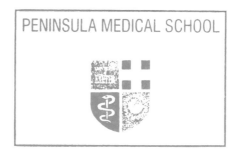

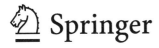 Springer

Editors
Carla M. Pugh
Department of Surgery
University of Wisconsin School
of Medicine and Public Health
Madison
Wisconsin, WI
USA

Rebecca S. Sippel
Department of Surgery
University of Wisconsin School
of Medicine and Public Health
Madison
Wisconsin, WI
USA

ISBN 978-1-4471-4690-2   ISBN 978-1-4471-4691-9   (eBook)
DOI 10.1007/978-1-4471-4691-9
Springer London Heidelberg New York Dordrecht

Library of Congress Control Number: 2013944893

Printed on acid-free paper

Springer is part of Springer Science+Business Media (www.springer.com)

To all of the educational leaders, role models, and mentors that have given their time, shared their passion, and painted a vision for the future

Acknowledgments

We would like to thank Dr. Herbert Chen and Dr. Lillian Kao and the AAS for inviting us to coordinate this project and Stephanie Olivas for her administrative support.

Contents

Contributors

Amalia Cochran, MD Department of Surgery, University of Utah,
Salt Lake City, UT, USA

Gary Dunnington, MD, FACS Department of Surgery, Indiana University
School of Medicine, Indianapolis, IN, USA

Liane S. Feldman, MD Division of General Surgery, McGill University
Health Centre, Montreal, QC, Canada

Gerald M. Fried, MD Department of Surgery, McGill University,
Montreal, QC, Canada

Heidi Gibbs, CPA, MBA Department of Surgery, Indiana University School of
Medicine, Indianapolis, IN, USA

Steven B. Goldin, MD, PhD Department of Surgery, University of South Florida,
Tampa General Hospital, Tampa, FL, USA

Jon C. Gould, MD Department of Surgery, Medical College of Wisconsin,
Milwaukee, WI, USA

Jacob A. Greenberg, MD, EdM Department of Surgery,
University of Wisconsin School of Medicine and Public Health,
Madison, WI, USA

Brandon V. Henry, MD, MPh Department of Surgery, Duke University
Medical Center, Durham, NC, USA

Gregory T. Horn, BA Department of Surgery, University of South Florida
Morsani College of Medicine, Tampa, FL, USA

Sinan Jabori Division of Vascular Surgery, UCLA Gonda (Goldschmied)
Vascular Center, David Geffen School of Medicine at UCLA,
Los Angeles, CA, USA

Roger H. Kim, MD Department of Surgery, Louisiana State University Health Sciences Center in Shreveport, Shreveport, LA, USA

Sara Kim, PhD Department of Surgery, Institute of Simulation and Interprofessional Studies (ISIS), School of Medicine, University of Washington, Seattle, WA, USA

Brenessa Lindeman, MD Department of Surgery, The Johns Hopkins Medical Institutions, Baltimore, MD, USA

Rebecca M. Minter, MD Department of Surgery, University of Michigan Health System, Ann Arbor, MI, USA

Paul N. Montero, MD Department of Surgery, University of Colorado School of Medicine, Aurora, CO, USA

Carlos A. Pellegrini, MD, FACS, FRCSI (Hon.) Department of Surgery, School of Medicine, University of Washington, Seattle, WA, USA

Jacob R. Peschman, MD Department of Surgery, Medical College of Wisconsin, Milwaukee, WI, USA

Roy Phitayakorn, MD, MHPE (MEd) Department of Surgery, The Massachusetts General Hospital, Harvard Medical School, Boston, MA, USA

Carla M. Pugh, MD, PhD Department of Surgery, University of Wisconsin School of Medicine and Public Health, Madison, WI, USA

Christopher D. Raeburn, MD, FACS Department of Surgery, University of Colorado School of Medicine, Aurora, CO, USA

C. Max Schmidt, MD, PhD, MBA, FACS Department of Surgery, Indiana University School of Medicine, Indianapolis, IN, USA

Rebecca S. Sippel, MD Department of Surgery, University of Wisconsin School of Medicine and Public Health, Madison, WI, USA

Dimitrios Stefanidis, MD, PhD, FACS Department of Surgery, Carolinas Simulation Center, Carolinas Healthcare System, Charlotte, NC, USA

Ranjan Sudan, MD Department of Surgery, Duke University Medical Center, Durham, NC, USA

Nicholas R. Teman, MD Department of Surgery, University of Michigan Health System, Ann Arbor, MI, USA

Laura Torbeck, PhD Department of Surgery, Indiana University School of Medicine, Indianapolis, IN, USA

Melina C. Vassiliou, MD, MED Department of Surgery, McGill University, Montreal, QC, Canada

Meghana Vellanki, BS Department of Medicine, University of South Florida, Morsani College of Medicine, Windermere, FL, USA

Stephen C. Yang, MD Department of Surgery, The Johns Hopkins Medical Institutions, Baltimore, MD, USA

Chapter 1
An Overview of Opportunities in Surgical Education

Rebecca S. Sippel and Carla M. Pugh

Background

The Past

Surgical education is part of the core mission of any department of surgery. The traditional view of surgical education largely focuses on teaching medical students and residents. In addition, leadership in surgical education was thought of as a stepping stone to other leadership positions within the department, training in education or teaching was not required, and it was thought that anyone was capable of being a surgical educator.

Educational Challenges

Increasing regulations, work-hour restrictions, and an increase emphasis on outcomes have created a need within departments for faculty that are not only "good" teachers but understand the issues confronting surgical education and can develop and run a competency-based surgical curriculum that not only exposes students and residents to the field of surgery but ensures that they are learning the core knowledge and skills that they need to be competent physicians and surgeons. No longer is it acceptable to simply "see one, do one, teach one."

R.S. Sippel, MD (✉) • C.M. Pugh, MD, PhD
Department of Surgery,
University of Wisconsin School of Medicine and Public Health,
Madison, WI, USA
e-mail: sippel@surgery.wisc.edu; pugh@surgery.wisc.edu

C.M. Pugh, R.S. Sippel (eds.), *Success in Academic Surgery:*
Developing a Career in Surgical Education, Success in Academic Surgery,
DOI 10.1007/978-1-4471-4691-9_1, © Springer-Verlag London 2013

The Evolving State of Surgical Education

Historically to be successful in surgery, each individual strived to be a "triple threat": an outstanding clinician, researcher, and teacher. While the concept of a triple threat has not disappeared, increasingly department chairs are recognizing that these are three core missions of the department, not necessarily of individual surgeons. The department as a whole needs to excel in each of these areas. In order to excel in education, there is a need to set evidence-based goals and commit to important infrastructure that educators need (training, time, and resources). As such there is a growing need for surgeons with not only an interest in surgical education, but also the training and expertise to help develop and support the educational mission of the department.

Success in surgical education cannot be accomplished alone. Educational programs need adequate administrative support and protected time for its administrators. Research programs need collaborators with expertise in education research. Increasingly departments of surgery are recognizing the need for PhD educators within the department to help fulfill and support these roles.

The Path to Becoming a Surgical Educator

Surgical education is a rapidly growing field with a variety of opportunities available to get involved. Due to this growth there is a critical need for surgeons with an interest and expertise in surgical education. For those of you that are interested in potentially making education your career focus, our hope is that this book will help to open your mind to some of the many possibilities available within the field of surgical education.

The first step to developing a career in surgical education is to get the correct training. For some people that will include pursuing an advanced degree either during residency or in their early years on faculty (see Chap. 11). But for many, taking the time to get an additional degree may not be feasible, and there are many other training opportunities available both within your institution and nationally that can help you to develop the skills you will need to be successful (see Chap. 10). In addition to getting the training that you need, you need to ensure that you can identify mentors that are supportive of your goal and can work with you to help you achieve them (see Chap. 9). For those of you that are interested in taking on leadership roles within your department in surgical education, it is essential to obtain skills in leadership (see Chap. 7) and an understanding of how the surgical education mission is financed (see Chap. 8).

Within the field of surgical education, there are a variety of opportunities to get involved. The two most common areas for involvement relate to medical student and resident teaching. While this includes being a clerkship director or a residency program director, there are a wealth of additional opportunities available in both the medical school and the graduate medical education office. Taking advantage of opportunities outside of the department can be a great opportunity for growth as a surgical educator. In Chaps. 2 and 3, we hope to highlight many of the unique opportunities available within these areas. Surgical simulation is a rapidly growing field, and surgeons are ideally suited to get involved in and to take on leadership roles within an institution's simulation center (see Chap. 4). Looking beyond the training years, there is an ever-increasing need for people with an expertise in continuing medical education, helping to address the needs of practicing surgeons with both maintenance of skills and knowledge as well as the acquisition of new skills once in practice.

In order to establish yourself as a surgical educator, it is important to get involved not only locally but also nationally in surgical education. There are many great opportunities to get involved at a national level which are highlighted in Chap. 5. Surgical education is an increasingly viable career path for promotion within academic surgery, but it is important that you understand the metrics for which you will be measured. Tips for how the process works and how to get promoted as a surgical educator are highlighted in Chap. 6.

Finding Your Niche and Succeeding at It

Once you have chosen your path, there must be a strategy involved in honing and defining your niche. Whether you choose to focus on undergraduate medical education, graduate medical education, or continuing medical education, additional work is necessary in defining your focus within these areas. Specific examples include a focus on curriculum development, program evaluation, performance assessment, or even specific clinical contexts. The opportunities are broad. The formal process of goal setting has been well defined and there are several strategies and approaches. The SMART concept states that your goals should be (1) *S*pecific, (2) *M*easureable, (3) *A*ttainable, (4) *R*ewarding, and (5) *T*imely.

Using the SMART concept, if your passion is simulation-based curriculum development for residents, it is recommended that you go through the process of writing down the following: What you wish to develop and what technology, content, financial support, and personal time are needed (Specific); how you will measure the success of your new curricula (Measurable); do you have the infrastructure including departmental support and key collaborators (Attainable); will you enjoy the work after noting the pros and cons of the work process (Rewarding); and can the goal be achieved in a reasonable time period without losing usefulness (Timely). Similarly, the SMART concept can be used in setting goals for obtaining local and national leadership positions.

The last section of this book has four chapters dealing with research in surgical education. This topic deserves special attention as it is pertinent to success regardless of your niche area. Use of qualitative or quantitative research methods to evaluate your program or execute specific experimental protocols will help to better define your goals and your niche. Publishing your work will help to build collaborations, establish local and national presence, and serve as the groundwork for obtaining funding.

Special Considerations

Graduate Study

It is extremely important to be aligned and mentored by a successful surgeon scientist during your graduate studies if you choose this route. Obtaining a Master's or PhD in education is a great step towards defining your career as educational leader however; it is uncommon for faculty and leadership in a school of education to understand the many nuances of surgical education. Moreover, it is unlikely that faculty in a school of education will know which societies you should plan to be involved in or where to present and publish your work. Lastly, if you are planning a research career in surgical education, it is critical to have an understanding of the tight balance that must be achieved when trying to succeed in a combined clinical and research position.

Ethics in Education Research

The worst outcome of any education research project is to leave the participants feeling that they were just a number and the exercise they just participated in was not useful because there was no feedback. This phenomenon is not special to research in surgical education, and there is an extensive amount of historical and new research regarding this in traditional education literature and peer-reviewed journals.

Bridging the Gap

In the process of achieving our professional goals in surgical education, we must be reminded of the gap that exists between actual practice and the results of our research. Feedback is one of the key elements that may facilitate bridging the gap. For example, if you studied the validity and reliability of a checklist for laparoscopic colectomy, this would require you to not only document correct and incorrect answers but also generate an understanding of how the incorrect answers should be built into focused learning or deliberate practice for the individual surgeon.

Quality and Patient Safety

While the ultimate goal is to develop educational systems and processes that benefit the patient, we have ways to go in developing and achieving goals that consistently drive successful quality and patient safety agendas. Outcomes and health services research have many direct links to education and collaborative initiatives that will be the key to achieving high-quality care.

Summary

In summary, the goal of the book is to provide an overview of important topics that must be considered when planning a successful career in surgical education. The three main sections of this book include: (1) Local and National Leadership Opportunities, (2) Professional Development, and (3) Research. All of the chapters have been written or coauthored by members of the Association for Academic Surgery (AAS), a premier organization for surgeon scientists.

Chapter 2
Opportunities in Medical Student Education

Brandon V. Henry and Ranjan Sudan

Abbreviations

AAS	Association for Academic Surgery
ACS	American College of Surgeons
AERA	American Educational Research Association
ASE	Association for Surgical Education
CD	Clerkship Director
CDs	Clerkship Directors
CESERT	Center for Excellence in Surgical Education, Research and Training
NBME	National Board of Medical Examiners

Introduction

Historically, medical education has been associated with a lengthy, intense, and demanding course of training requiring much sacrifice on the part of the trainee. After 12 years of high school and 4 years of college, the aspiring physician spends an additional 4 years in medical school before spending a minimum of 5 more years of residency training in surgery. This duration can be prolonged by significant length for those pursuing research and/or subspecialty training.

Every year the American Association of Medical Colleges conducts a survey of graduating medical students to evaluate their medical school experience (GQ medical student graduation questionnaire), and in the 2011 survey, work-life

B.V. Henry, MD, MPH • R. Sudan, MD (✉)
Department of Surgery, Duke University Medical Center,
Durham, NC 27710, USA
e-mail: brandon.henry@duke.edu; ranjan.sudan@duke.edu

C.M. Pugh, R.S. Sippel (eds.), *Success in Academic Surgery:*
Developing a Career in Surgical Education, Success in Academic Surgery,
DOI 10.1007/978-1-4471-4691-9_2, © Springer-Verlag London 2013

balance was listed by students as having a strong influence on their career choice. This number increased from 37 % in 2009 to 43.3 % in 2011. If this trend continues, many students may not pursue surgery due to its very lengthy training track. However, 81.9 % of the students rated content of a specialty and 86.7 % rated fit of personality, interests, and skills as strong influences on a career choice. While surgeon educators may not be able to influence a personality fit, we definitely have the ability to improve the content and teach technical skills and thereby increase the interest of students in our field. In fact, if we are to encourage the best and the brightest to join our field, become our trainees and subsequently our peers and caregivers, then it is imperative that we show them the best side of surgery.

We can recognize and understand some of the existing opportunities to interact and influence medical students in a positive manner from the 2011 GQ questionnaire. For instance, in 2009 about a third of the students either disagreed or strongly disagreed with a statement that surgery faculty members had observed them perform a history or a physical examination (on a Likert scale of 1–5, with 1 being strongly disagree and 5 as strongly agree). The mean score for a surgery faculty member observing history taking was 3.3 and the mean score for observing physical examination was 3.4. On the surface these scores do not appear particularly disappointing until they are compared with the scores of internal medicine faculty who scored 4.0 and 4.1, respectively. Surgery faculty also scored lower compared to internal medicine faculty and even surgery residents when providing feedback to students (mean score 3.7 vs. 4.2 and 4.1, respectively). The scores for providing feedback to students had a very similar distribution to that of direct clinical observation of students. Due to the changing practice environment, time has become a precious commodity for surgery faculty and is being reflected in these lower scores. The fact that surgery residents were rated higher than surgery faculty in observing history and physicals indicates that the education and well-being of medical students in surgery have shifted from being the primary responsibility of faculty to that of the residents. Since residents are in constant contact with the students, it is understandable that residents play a major role in student education. However, surgery faculty should not underestimate their own importance as role models. In the same questionnaire 77 % of the students felt that role models either moderately or strongly influenced their career choice. The students valued role models higher than competitiveness of a specialty, degree of indebtedness, or ability to generate income from a specialty choice [1].

The bright side to the story in surgery is that most surgeons love their work. They perform technical miracles every day and turn pure misery into instant relief for many of their patients. The hopes and dreams of many patients and their families and their very survival rest in the hands of surgeons. Patients are enormously grateful to their surgeons and this gratitude brings much job satisfaction. This is part of what makes being a surgeon so great and we must share this positive side of surgery with our students. This chapter is dedicated towards helping surgeon educators understand the wonderful opportunities that exist in medical education but, more importantly, to help every surgeon understand that each interaction with a student is an opportunity to impact their perception of the field of surgery. In fact, the absence of interaction is often viewed by students as neglect and can be just as devastating as a negative interaction. Perceptions and interest in surgical careers can improve after exposure to surgical clerkships. Hence, the responsibility of portraying surgery in a positive light rests on the shoulders of all those who have chosen surgery as their profession. The message is simple. As surgeon educators we need to be spending more time interacting with students. This can be accomplished, in part, by observing students perform their day-to-day clinical work and by providing immediate feedback on their performance.

In order to help surgeons become knowledgeable about opportunities in medical student education, it is helpful to create a framework that encompasses the medical student curriculum through all 4 years of medical school. Curriculum can broadly be divided into three types. The first is the formal curriculum. This has an organized structure and consists of activities such as lectures, group discussions, and the simulation laboratory. The formal curriculum may not be the best form of learning because it is non-contextual, but it is a necessary means of covering certain subject material in a time-efficient manner. It also provides uniform instruction across multiple sites and lends itself to testing and evaluations. The informal curriculum refers to more opportunistic learning that is contextual and is taught in a mentorship model such as on the floor, in the operating room, or when interesting clinical material presents itself. Finally, the hidden curriculum is the unwritten code of expectations by which members of a profession behave within their environment [2]. Faculty members can participate in all of these curricula at either the departmental level, within the medical school, or both. Opportunities to participate in education also exist at the national level through education societies (Association for Surgical Education) or specialty societies that have dedicated sections for medical students at their annual meeting (American College of Surgeons or the Association for Academic Surgery). In order to facilitate professional development either as an educator or researcher, a partial list of teaching opportunities and resources is included in Tables 2.1 and 2.2.

Departmental Opportunities

Clerkship Director (CD)

Clerkship directors (CDs) play a central role in setting the tone for the core clerkship at the third-year level. Their responsibilities include developing the goals and objectives, the content that helps meet these, and evaluations of the students for the medical school. CDs also select faculty who participate in the curriculum. The surgical clerkships can influence medical student perceptions of surgical career options [3]. This limited period of time—as short as 6 weeks in some schools—can often become a considerable determinant in whether a student pursues or turns away from a future in surgical practice. As a CD, one can create a learning environment

Table 2.1 Opportunities for involvement in medical student education

Direct interaction—preclinical (years 1–2)
Anatomy laboratory instruction
Didactic clinical correlations for basic science subjects
Clinical shadowing
Research project involvement
Individual mentoring
Surgical interest group advising
Direct interaction—clinical/clerkship (years 3–4)
Clinic/operative instruction
Didactic/case presentation sessions
Small group discussion and debates
Basic skills/simulation training
Individual mentorship
Residency application/interview preparation
Pre-internship training workshops/boot camp
Administrative/curriculum development roles
Vice Dean of Education
Associate Dean of Education
Curriculum Committee/Advisory Board Member
Surgical Clerkship/Sub-internship Director
Department Chair (Chief)
Department Vice/Associate Chair
Residency Program Director
National society roles
American College of Surgeons Committee on Education
The Association for Surgical Education
The Association for Academic Surgery Education Committee
American Medical Association Council On Medical Education
Association of American Medical Colleges

Table 2.2 Career advancement and research opportunities/funding

Professional enrichment and advancement resources	Source[a]
Education Clearinghouse and PowerPoint Teaching Modules	ASE
Surgical Education Research Fellowship Program	ASE
Surgeons as Educators Course	ACS
Educational research funding	
Stemmler Medical Education Research Fund	NBME
Center for Excellence in Surgical Education, Research and Training (CESERT) Grants	ASE
Roslyn Faculty Research Award (Junior Faculty)	AAS
American Educational Research Association Grants	AERA
Individual Home Institution Innovation or GME Grants	Varies
Association for the Study of Medical Education Grants	ASME (UK)

[a]*ASE* the Association for Surgical Education, *ACS* American College of Surgeons, *NBME* National Board of Medical Examiners

that fosters interest in the field, disproves negative myths and stereotypes about surgeons, and provides a solid foundation of basic surgical knowledge for students regardless of their final career path.

The CD can seek out talented teaching faculty and residents to create engaging and informative didactic lessons and generate effective clinical experiences. In addition, they can empower students to feel welcome and become involved in patient care. CDs have access to a wide variety of surveys from students, house staff, and faculty that can be utilized to assist in reviewing the educational environment of the clerkship. As student attitudes and expectations may fluctuate from year to year, the CD can act as an effective liaison between students and faculty educators to continually enhance the experience for all. The CD functions as a guide or facilitator for students interested in surgical careers, and by being approachable and accessible, the director can point students towards appropriate surgical mentors. Also, the CD works in concert with the residency program director to increase resident involvement in the clerkship curriculum. In many institutions the CD may additionally supervise the clinical electives or sub-internships in year four of medical school, but in some instances, a different faculty member may have this responsibility.

It is estimated that CDs require 25 % of protected time for administrative responsibilities and 25 % additional time for hands-on teaching by the Alliance for Clinical Education [4]. In addition, a full-time clerkship coordinator is recommended.

Often the job of a CD falls to a relatively junior faculty member who is a relatively inexperienced educator and faces additional pressures to develop a clinical practice and research for their own academic growth. Under these circumstances it takes great discipline to maintain balance and protect time for educational responsibilities and growth as an educator. This is also a great opportunity for a younger faculty member to gain recognition in the medical school by participating in various committees such as the Curriculum Committee, the Promotions Committee, and the Admissions Committee. In order to help advance their professional development, the weeklong Surgeons as Educators Course, provided by the American College of Surgeons (ACS), is a very good resource. The Association for Surgical Education (ASE) is dedicated to advancing education in surgery and, through its Clerkship Directors Committee, offers courses specific to CDs. The job of a CD can be very gratifying as well as academically rewarding. About 95 % of CDs report enhanced job satisfaction and 70 % perceive it having a positive effect on their academic career [5].

Chairman

The Chair (or Chief) of a surgical department conveys the overall expectation of dedication to teaching to staff and surgical trainees. By making a dedicated effort to directly teach students, whether in the clinic, wards, or formalized didactic settings, the Chair can set the tone for what is expected of others. Formal teaching requirements and recognition can be set to ensure faculty participation in the medical school curriculum. In addition, the Chair can identify particularly enthusiastic and talented teaching faculty and encourage them to become closely involved in curriculum development and implementation.

The Chair controls the resources that support the teaching efforts of the CD and surgical faculty. Often, in tough economic times, teaching budgets can get cut. It has been shown that financial rewards are helpful but recognition for teaching efforts may be just as important for motivating faculty to participate in teaching [6]. By protecting teaching time for faculty and supporting academic advancement and recognition, the Chair can support the educational mission both in words and in deeds.

Vice/Associate Chair of Education

This role is becoming more common in institutions and can be fulfilled by either a surgeon or a PhD or EdD educator. The job description varies within each institution and is typically negotiated with the Chair of the department. Such negotiations typically cover protected time, principal areas of responsibility, and salary. Broadly, this individual's role is to provide guidance to the clerkship directors and program directors and interact with other programs in a cross departmental role. They are generally more seasoned educators and typically are more senior faculty members.

Residency Program Leadership

A program director is mostly occupied running a surgery residency program. However, much of the daily clinical instruction that students receive is generated through interactions with surgical trainees. Therefore, it is critically important that surgical residents actively engage in the education of medical students. Doing so improves the student experience, lays the groundwork for residents to become willing and effective clinical teachers throughout their careers, and positively impacts student perceptions of the field. This can serve to generate interest in the pursuit of further surgical training among students. The residency program director (or other formal participants in training program leadership) can greatly influence positive interaction between students and surgical residents. With guidance and motivation, surgical residents can become effective educators and mentors for medical students [7]. The program director can expect and require resident participation in student education on the wards and in the operating rooms. They can also work with the CD to facilitate resident interaction with students by creating protected time for residents to be involved in didactic teaching sessions and basic surgical skills training.

The program director also serves an important advisory role for medical students interested in applying to surgical residency training programs. A medical student is more likely to rate their home institution higher in the residency match if they have had a positive interaction with the program director. Therefore, arranging periodic didactic or case presentation sessions with prospective surgical trainees and students rotating through the surgical clerkships is a wonderful opportunity to create this interaction. Participation in student surgical interest group (SIG) events will provide even more opportunities to interact with students. Active program director involvement will enhance the students' educational experience, generate further interest in surgery, and be of aid when they apply for residency positions.

Medical School Committee/Leadership Opportunities

Surgical educators can seek involvement in medical student education via administrative positions within the Office of Curriculum/Curricular Affairs. Senior staff positions such as Vice Dean of Education and Associate Dean of Education can have a great amount of influence on the magnitude of emphasis on surgical education within the overall curriculum. Obtaining such positions can be an invaluable opportunity for a passionate surgical educator. One should also seek out positions on available curriculum advisory boards or within the faculty senate as these are good opportunities to interact with educators from other departments and learn best practices. Being on the admissions committee is an honor and a service to the institution. By helping select great applicants, it is easy to set the stage for success.

National Opportunities

The Association for Surgical Association (ASE) is the premier organization to become engaged in medical student education at the national level. Through its annual meeting, surgeon educators can learn about innovative methods of education and the latest in educational research and can participate in a variety of programs designed for professional growth such as the Surgical Education Research Fellowship (SERF). It has an open committee structure that is welcoming of member participation. Participation in the society allows surgeon educators to impact medical student education policy via the Committee on Curriculum. The Clerkship Directors Committee is a good resource for professional growth and networking with other clerkship directors. The American College of Surgeons (ACS) and the Association for Academic Surgery (AAS) also have robust medical student programs at their annual meetings and are a good forum to present research conducted by medical students. Funding to conduct research in medical education is available through a variety of grant programs and a partial list is included in Table 2.2.

Teaching Opportunities (Formal and Informal Curriculum)

These are opportunities that are open to all surgery faculty members and are divided by year of medical school for convenience.

Years 1–2 (Basic Science/Classroom Years)

Multiple opportunities exist to begin the surgical education of medical students during their first 2 years of study. Most medical school curriculums include human anatomy courses early in student coursework. The importance of understanding anatomy is essential for building a good foundation for learning in surgical practice. The anatomy laboratory setting can be used to assist students with cadaveric dissections to teach basic anatomical concepts. This also gives students their first glimpse into how a surgeon identifies and isolates important structures. This early interaction can encourage the formation of mentoring relationships between involved faculty and each new class of students.

Presentations by surgeons that are adjunct to the basic science curriculum are an opportunity to creatively introduce the role of surgical management in various disease states. This adds relevance and interest to the dryness of the basic science topics and places the role of surgery in its proper perspective. Surgical educators should be involved in core curriculum development to ensure that these opportunities are not missed. Arrangements for these activities can be made through the medical school Office of Curriculum.

Shadowing/Research Opportunities for Years 1–2

Many first- and second-year students are interested in clinical shadowing experiences, and some medical schools even require students to spend time shadowing physicians in the hospital during the basic science years. This presents a great opportunity for faculty to interact with students and show them real-life surgery before they have made up their minds about a certain specialty. Observing surgical practice in the clinics and operating rooms early may increase interest in the field of surgery among younger students who may have had little prior exposure. By providing a list of names to the medical school, students can be made aware of the surgeons who are interested in having students shadow them. Students should also be made aware of and encouraged to attend public surgical presentations (e.g., grand rounds, visiting professor lectures). Surgical educators can further interact with students by working together on research projects. This collaboration benefits students by providing valuable opportunities to conduct medical research and also builds important mentoring relationships that can last for the rest of the medical school experience and beyond.

Years 3–4 (Clerkships/Sub-internships)

The third- and fourth-year clinical rotations are critically important to the surgical education of medical students. Under the guidance of the surgical clerkship director, students will spend months at a time in operating rooms, outpatient clinics, and inpatient units helping in the care of surgical patients. There are many opportunities for surgical educators to teach and influence students during this period. It is very important that preceptors actively engage the students in hands-on teaching on the clinical services. Much can be learned simply by observation, but active involvement in patient care will create a much more enriching and memorable experience.

Surgical educators can teach basic surgical skills in multiple ways. Prior to entering the operating room, students can be taught basic suturing, knot tying, cutting, and other skills in a low-intensity setting rather than the more stressful real-time experience under the bright lights of the operating room. Programs with appropriate resources may attempt to implement simulator training sessions for upper-level medical students as well such as laparoscopic camera management simulation. As students progress from the core clerkship into their sub-internships, they can become increasingly involved in operative procedures. Actively engaging the students in closing skin incisions and assisting with simple portions of dissection under attending supervision will enhance skill development and engender greater interest in surgery.

In addition to clinical and operative instruction, surgical educators can participate in didactic teaching sessions and case presentation sessions with medical students. This can be accomplished either as part of the formal clerkship curriculum or during breaks in daily clinical duties. Individually engaging students in discussions or brief presentations on various key subjects further encourages teaching interaction.

Some institutions have dedicated surgery "boot camp" to prepare senior-level medical students for a surgery residency. Utilizing simulation materials, students can be introduced to more advanced skills such as complex suture techniques, placement of central lines, endotracheal tubes, and chest tubes. Basic laparoscopic techniques can be taught using virtual simulators and box trainers when available. Common surgical ward patient care issues and emergencies can be reviewed to help prepare these students for their surgical internship. Dictating operative notes and computerized order entry are also frequently taught.

Teaching Opportunities (Hidden Curriculum)

The hidden curriculum can be thought of as the culture of the specialty in a particular institution. Much of this is implicit and learning takes place by observing the behavior of others or by observing the response of authority figures to deviations of the norm. This is where faculty members can become good role models and set the tone for a positive environment in surgery. If all that the students heard was long hours, impending inefficiencies with electronic medical records, administrative challenges, declining reimbursement, and difficult patients, the students are unlikely to get excited about surgery. Such "recreational complaining" is common but has a deleterious effect on those sharing the conversation. Another disappointment for students is not being actively engaged in teaching by faculty in the operating room or in the clinics and wards. This neglect makes students feel unwanted and they do not like or admire people who make them feel so. Lack of admiration and respect will make it unlikely that a student will want to follow in their footsteps. On the other hand, if students are able to participate in the faculty's joy at the end of a case well done, the excitement that surgeons have coming to work every day, the satisfaction of obtaining an interesting titbit of knowledge that they did not previously have, and are made to feel that faculty are interested in their education, then it is quite likely that students would see surgery as a positive environment. If they witness verbally abusive faculty towards residents or staff, they will either be turned off or learn to repeat such unacceptable behavior. Neither is desirable. On the other hand, if students experience professionalism in interactions, then faculty will earn their respect and students will see them as positive role models who they hope to emulate. This is the hidden curriculum and each faculty member has the opportunity to educate students in achieving and maintaining high standards in this way [2, 8, 9].

Mentoring Opportunities/Surgery Interest Groups

Effective faculty mentorship should begin early for students planning to pursue surgical careers. Faculty members should make themselves available as advisors for interested students and present them with opportunities that will increase their exposure to the field. In particular, the surgical clerkship director and residency program director can act as easily identifiable liaisons for these students, guiding them towards appropriate individual mentors. Surgical educators can also provide mentorship by becoming involved in surgery interest groups (SIGs). They can also facilitate involvement of other faculty in events related to the SIG and be a resource for general advice to participating students. In fact, many SIGs invite faculty and residents to speak about a range of topics from how to prepare for residency to a particular surgeon's area of research. The ASE provides helpful information about starting a SIG and the role of a faculty advisor in such groups [10].

As students draw closer to the residency application process, effective mentors will show students how to maximize the yield of each of their rotations by suggesting study materials and emphasizing which elements of clinical rotations to focus upon. Mentors can also suggest research projects and useful extracurricular activities for students. Assistance with application review and interview preparation will be useful services that mentors can provide during the application process. In addition, involved surgical mentors, through their own personal example, demonstrate to these budding surgical trainees that providing education and mentoring for students is an important and necessary responsibility that should be embraced by all.

Table 2.3 Necessary components of intellectual development statement for promotions and tenure

A brief biographical history including educational background
Documentation of clinical and research activities
Teaching contributions which include accomplishments and plans as a teacher, mentor, and educator
Personal goals and strategies for meeting them
Tabular summary of teaching and mentoring activities (by year)
Academic achievements and scholarship
Grant support
Leadership (local, national, and international)
Institutional service
Vision and plans for continued professional growth and development in an academic environment

(Per Duke University 2013)

Career Advancement Opportunities

In most academic institutions, there are designated clinician-teacher tracks and active engagement in teaching has become a bona fide route for career advancement [11]. This often requires the creation of a teaching portfolio. Each institution has its own requirements, and it is a good idea for educators to familiarize themselves with the documentation early because they are often extensive and difficult to recreate in retrospect. Either the faculty handbook or the Office of Academic Affairs can assist in understanding these requirements. An example of the contents of an intellectual development statement from an academic institution is included in Table 2.3. Besides academic advancement, being engaged in teaching can be very fulfilling on a personal level.

Conclusion

Many opportunities exist for surgical educators to become closely involved in the education of medical students. The clerkship experience represents the most focused period of surgical study for students and can be greatly influential as they begin to make career decisions. In addition to being enthusiastically involved in the clerkships, surgical educators can participate in several other aspects of medical education. Early in the basic science curriculum, surgeons can assist in presenting clinical correlations and proctor practical lab sessions. Surgeons can be effective mentors with regard to both clinical and research endeavors. Educators have the ability to influence students greatly through direct guidance and demonstrated behavior. Furthermore, administrative influence can serve to enhance the opportunities for medical students to interact with surgeons and obtain valuable exposures to the field. These experiences can include, but are not limited to, clinical shadowing, attending departmental conferences, individual mentoring, and simulated surgical skills training. Enthusiasm and creativity should be employed to ensure the best possible basic surgical training for our future physicians, regardless of their eventual chosen specialty. Such an experience is gratifying for both the students and the educators.

References

1. Medical Student Graduation Questionnaire. 2011. Available from: https://www.aamc.org/data/gq/. Cited 27 July 2012.
2. Gofton W, Regehr G. What we don't know we are teaching: unveiling the hidden curriculum. Clin Orthop Relat Res. 2006;449:20–7. Epub 2006/06/01.
3. O'Herrin JK, Lewis BJ, Rikkers LF, Chen H. Why do students choose careers in surgery? J Surg Res. 2004;119(2):124–9. Epub 2004/05/18.
4. Pangaro L, Bachicha J, Brodkey A, Chumley-Jones H, Fincher RM, Gelb D, et al. Expectations of and for clerkship directors: a collaborative statement from the Alliance for Clinical Education. Teach Learn Med. 2003;15(3):217–22.
5. Ephgrave K, Ferguson K, Shaaban A, Hoshi H. Resources and rewards for clerkship directors: how surgery compares. Am J Surg. 2010;199(1):66–71. Epub 2010/01/28.
6. Williams RG, Dunnington GL, Folse JR. The impact of a program for systematically recognizing and rewarding academic performance. Acad Med. 2003;78(2):156–66. Epub 2003/02/14.
7. Musunuru S, Lewis B, Rikkers LF, Chen H. Effective surgical residents strongly influence medical students to pursue surgical careers. J Am Coll Surg. 2007;204(1):164–7. Epub 2006/12/26.
8. Hunt DD, Scott C, Zhong S, Goldstein E. Frequency and effect of negative comments ("badmouthing") on medical students' career choices. Acad Med. 1996;71(6):665–9. Epub 1996/06/01.
9. Rogers DA, Boehler ML, Roberts NK, Johnson V. Using the hidden curriculum to teach professionalism during the surgery clerkship. J Surg Educ. 2012;69(3):423–7. Epub 2012/04/10.
10. Surgery Interest Groups. Association for Surgical Education. 2012. Available from: http://ase.memberclicks.net/sig-overview. Cited 30 July 2012.
11. Sanfey H, Gantt NL. Career development resource: academic career in surgical education. Am J Surg. 2012;204(1):126–9. Epub 2012/06/19.

Chapter 3
Opportunities in Resident Education

Paul N. Montero and Christopher D. Raeburn

One of the most compelling reasons for choosing the field of medicine is the ability to help others, and this altruistic drive is common to the field of education. In fact, the word *doctor* is derived from the Latin root *docēre* – to teach. Thus, it is not surprising that many physicians find the combination of healing and education to be incredibly gratifying. This chapter will describe a variety of considerations for surgeon educators including: (1) benefits and barriers to surgical education, (2) opportunities for teaching surgical residents, and (3) opportunities for career advancement in surgical education.

Teaching is the highest form of understanding.

– Aristotle

Anyone who has ever prepared for and given a talk to surgical residents knows what Aristotle was talking about; there is no better way to determine ones understanding of a topic than to attempt to teach it. What better way for a faculty member to stay abreast of the current literature on a surgical topic (and prepare for recertification exams!) than to actively prepare for and administer a teaching session for the residents? While this type of teaching opportunity may directly benefit the faculty, there are a multitude of other opportunities for the surgical educator where the incentive may be less obvious but the reward just as gratifying. For instance, spending the extra time to safely take an intern through a laparoscopic cholecystectomy can (at times) be more satisfying to a faculty member than had they just done the case themselves. More important, however, is that the impact of that experience on the intern can be enormous. Indeed, it has been said that the true greatness of a surgeon is measured not merely by the number of patients they benefited but by the number of good surgeons he or she has helped train.

P.N. Montero, MD • C.D. Raeburn, MD, FACS (✉)
Department of Surgery,
University of Colorado School of Medicine,
Aurora, CO, USA
e-mail: christopher.raeburn@ucdenver.edu; paul.montero@ucdenver.edu

C.M. Pugh, R.S. Sippel (eds.), *Success in Academic Surgery:*
Developing a Career in Surgical Education, Success in Academic Surgery,
DOI 10.1007/978-1-4471-4691-9_3, © Springer-Verlag London 2013

Just as there are diverse opportunities for faculty to participate in research within a department, so are there a myriad opportunities for participating in education. Not all surgical faculty will have the same level of commitment to resident education nor will they all possess the same strengths, but the vast majority of academic faculty, at some level, enjoy and benefit by working in a teaching environment. To build and maintain a strong educational program, residency programs should systematically "take inventory" of their teaching faculty and carefully allocate and cultivate those faculty for specific educational purposes. For instance, some faculty might not be best suited for formal didactic teaching sessions but instead might have excellent operative teaching skills. Recognizing this, the program might build upon the strengths of those faculty by contributing resources to make instructional operative videos or having them facilitate animal labs. Having an assistant or associate program director whose main responsibility is surgical education is vital to this process. This person can assess the educational needs of the residents and the availability and teaching strengths of the faculty and then facilitate the program in developing strategies to meet those educational needs and appropriately direct resource support.

Effective teaching may be the hardest job there is.

– William Glasser

As Dr. Glasser points out, teaching is not necessarily easy, so it is understandable that not all surgeons choose to become surgical educators. Common barriers that might prevent an otherwise willing and able faculty member from participating in resident education include time burden, lack of direct financial compensation, lack of confidence, and lack of knowledge as to what opportunities for education exist. The combination of decreasing clinical reimbursement and rising regulatory requirements increasingly pressures faculty to spend more time in clinical activities. This impinges on what time faculty might otherwise be willing to commit to resident education. These same factors also decrease available funds that hospitals and departments have to financially compensate faculty who devote time and effort to education. In addition, most faculty have not had any formal training in education and, therefore, may feel that they are not qualified or may even feel intimidated about teaching. While it is ultimately the faculty member's individual decision to participate in surgical education, efforts by the department and program leadership to limit the above barriers are vital in promoting and maintaining a strong faculty commitment to surgical education.

Setting aside time to provide resident education may in itself be difficult, but corralling residents together in the same location for a period of time, free of patient care distractions, can often seem impossible. This is particularly true for residencies that encompass multiple hospital sites. It can be quite frustrating for faculty who devote the time to prepare for a teaching session only to have poor attendance by the residents and/or multiple distractions. Having protected time for didactic teaching and utilizing teleconferencing capabilities to synchronize that time across different hospital sites are a must. Optimal learning often encompasses digital media, audiovisual capabilities, or simulator technology. Acquisition of such amenities can be expensive or even prohibitive in the restricted budgets of surgical departments

Table 3.1 Obstacles and potential solutions to resident education

Obstacle	Potential solution
Time constraint	Effective planning
	Repeated small group lectures
	Resource utilization – prepackaged lectures, presentations, handouts
Cost constraint	Creativity, interdepartmental collaboration, grant funding, industry sponsorship
Location constraint	Web-based curricula, closed circuit televised lectures to satellite locations
Resident participation	Interaction – questions, hands-on approach, senior teaching roles Technology – audience response systems, videos, images
	Performance or knowledge-based goals
	Mandated participation/mandated protected time

Table 3.2 Resident stressors

Patient care – call, pages, notes, clinic, OR
Time constraints – work hours, clinic, discharges
Debt load – medical school, undergraduate, student loan payments, cost of living
Family – spouse, children, parents/siblings
Policies/technology – logging work hours, logging cases, electronic medical records, multiple computer access codes

nationwide. Table 3.1 lists several common obstacles to resident education and potential solutions to address them. An important role for the surgeon educator is in the recognition and resolution of these obstacles.

Surgical Education of Residents: *Who* You Are Teaching

In contrast to college and medical school, residency offers an entirely different structure and is accompanied by significant stressors and distractions (Table 3.2). First and foremost, residents have the immense responsibility of providing safe patient care during their training. The balance of education and patient care can be tedious and difficult to navigate. "Service versus education" is a constant source of debate and strain when allocating resources and seeking ACGME accreditation. Not surprisingly, residents, hospitals, and program directors often disagree on what entails service versus education. The surgeon educator can help bridge this gap by emphasizing teaching points during routine patient care.

Time management is increasingly more complex in the era of the 80-h workweek. Sophisticated shift schedules, frequent patient sign-out requirements, and intricate work-hour logging systems as well as electronic medical records can significantly cut into time for resident education. The surgical resident must carve out time for education in these complex schedules and adapt to each rotation accordingly. This highlights the need for organized and enthusiastic educators to assist in creating a streamlined learning process.

As opposed to the highly structured educational process of premedical and medical education, surgical residency education is more self-driven and self-paced. Gone are the organizational concepts of the syllabus, routine quizzes or tests, and reading requirements to which the learner has become accustomed and held accountable. This shift may be particularly challenging for *Generation Y* residents, who have been raised in a technology-dominated culture where information is instantly accessible, and committing details to memory may seem extraneous. The loss of this hierarchical and organized learning environment can be difficult and frustrating for residents who might have previously flourished but now find themselves struggling to adjust to the learning environment of residency. Having a formal mentoring system can be of great benefit in the early recognition of residents who may need additional help with this transition.

Indeed, surveys of surgical residents have demonstrated that the availability of a documented and structured training curriculum and routine teaching activities such as bedside teaching rounds and morbidity/mortality conferences strongly influence trainee satisfaction. A surgeon educator can help to improve the learning experience for residents by developing a standard curriculum specific to a certain service or rotation. While it will not be comprehensive, the curriculum might include a review of the common problems and operations encountered on that service, a list of learning objectives, selected readings, and expectations of the residents. Providing this structure and organization to a rotation gives the resident a framework on which to build knowledge and confidence.

By the time medical trainees enter residency, many have families and are faced with the requirement of student loan repayments while earning a modest stipend. Faced with the debt load from medical school and often undergraduate education, this can also be a significant source of stress. Aforementioned time constraints and patient care considerations also have the capacity to create significant stress for the surgical resident and his or her family outside of the hospital. The additive effect of these stressors can result in a downward spiral from which it is very difficult for a resident to recover. Here again, a mentor can be highly valuable in the early recognition of such a problem so that the resident can receive appropriate support from the program. While this may not seem like a role for a surgeon educator, until such residents receive the help that they need, their ability to learn will be severely impaired.

Finally, although human anatomy has remained constant (except for increasing habitus), today's surgical resident has a vastly increased fund of knowledge to acquire in comparison to those surgeons on the brink of retirement. The fields of laparoscopy, diagnostic and interventional radiology, endoscopy, oncology, and critical care are among the many areas of innovation and advancement that current residents must embrace. Evidence-based medicine continues to evolve exponentially and requires great effort to keep pace with, particularly amidst the nearly ubiquitous influences of industry marketing in the medical field. Further adding to this burden is the need to comply with ever-increasing regulatory requirements and master the use of complicated electronic medical records. Indeed, as residents often feel lucky to be able to even have lunch on any given day, it is no wonder that they

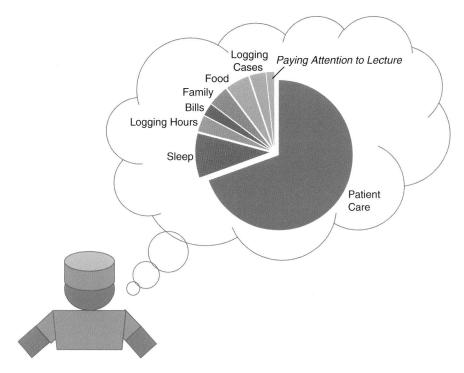

Fig. 3.1 What the resident is thinking about during your lecture

may find it difficult to set aside extracurricular time to read and learn (Fig. 3.1). In the current and complex work-hour restricted era, the responsibility of *effective* education falls to you, the surgeon educator.

Surgical Education of Residents: *Where* You Are Teaching

There are different learning environments for the resident surgeon, where balancing patient safety and satisfaction with resident participation and autonomy can be difficult. The operating room, surgery clinic, surgical ward, and classroom each provide unique opportunities for education.

The operating room is a challenging environment in which the surgeon educator must balance efficiency, patient safety, and resident proficiency and confidence. Resident preparation is paramount to effective operative education and should be encouraged and verified. Atlases, videos, and articles are available to assist the resident, and when possible, the surgeon educator's own notes, videos, or syllabus should be reviewed preoperatively. Additionally, several procedures have an associated cognitive task analysis (CTA) reported in the literature. This entails additional insight gained from interviews and observations of experts performing a task or procedure and incorporates strategies, decision-making algorithms, and key steps. CTA has been shown to enhance a surgical educator's instructions. Operative briefing and debriefing are important opportunities to review the surgical plan and ensure that appropriate understanding takes place. Close analysis of a resident's dictated operative report is an often overlooked opportunity to verify and improve their understanding of the procedure. Other assessment tools, such as the Global Operative Assessment of Laparoscopic Skills (GOALS), offer validated and feasible methods of providing structured feedback to the resident surgeon. Additionally, placing the resident in a teaching role for his or her junior resident is an excellent method of assessing their understanding of the procedure.

The surgery clinic also pits patient satisfaction and clinic workflow versus resident education, decision-making, and autonomy. It is also a realm where minimization of "scut work" and emphasis on education can help demonstrate to the resident the educational value of patient care over the "service" aspect. The astute resident should recognize the utility of clinic for commonly encountered patient questions or problems, styles of explanation and consent, the ability and technique of teaching patients, and interdepartmental communication/diplomacy skills (professionalism). Commonly used strategies for residents in clinic include shadowing the attending and seeing patients then presenting them. Emphasis should be placed on bedside teaching and concomitant evaluation, where the educator can pay attention to the resident's history acquisition and physical exam skills.

The patient wards also carry the challenges of patient safety and satisfaction, resident efficiency and autonomy, and minimization of "scut work." Time constraints generally prohibit collective rounds led by the attending, and a critical teaching and leadership opportunity for senior residents often ensues, unobserved by surgeon educators. This autonomy and lack of "micromanagement" is an integral part of resident education and confidence but needs oversight and input to maintain patient safety. This remains an area ripe for further research.

Finally, didactic lectures offer an imperfect yet effective opportunity to educate residents. Time and location constraints, attentiveness (i.e., post-call residents or patient care distractions), and educator effectiveness all impact the utility of such teaching sessions. Effective strategies include resident interaction, such as the use of a "mock orals" format; embracing technology such as operative images, audience response systems, and web-based resources; and selection of topics that residents request or that are not sufficiently discussed in textbooks or articles (such as electrosurgical instruments or surgical staplers).

Surgical Education of Residents: *Opportunities* for Teaching

When the learner, environment, and infrastructure of the program are carefully considered, subtle opportunities for resident teaching present themselves (Table 3.3) and must be captured by the surgeon educator. Other educational opportunities are less subtle. Although programs vary widely, each residency has didactic lectures, journal

Table 3.3 Educational opportunities in resident education

Substitute/guest lecturer in established didactic

Skills labs

Proctoring web-based curricula

Educational grants and research

Test preparation

Orientation/"boot camp"

Spontaneous educational presentations

Operative briefing/debriefing

Teaching rounds

clubs, grand rounds, and mortality and morbidity conferences that serve as the foundation of surgical education. These activities are often led by established surgeon educators in the program, but invariably the hectic schedules of academic surgeons will lead to opportunities during their absence. Those interested in surgical education can begin with participation in these established events. Tailoring topics to pertinent care issues or resident-requested topics can help garner resident interest and participation. Prospective surgeon educators should maintain teaching files of laparoscopic videos, intraoperative photos, radiology images, and unused surgical instruments to enhance these lectures. When applicable, a hands-on approach using central line kits, pieces of surgical mesh, or surgical staplers, for example, will augment the education.

Though more demanding of time and resources, surgical educators can also create educational opportunities such as skills lab sessions. Industry representatives are often willing to assist in organizing and financing these endeavors; however, this carries with it the responsibility of maintaining an unbiased educational atmosphere and adherence to institutional conflict of interest policies. Dry labs, vivariums, and cadaveric dissections are excellent vehicles to provide skills-based learning with reproducibility and structure and without patient safety concerns. The ubiquitous obstacle of resident participation in these labs can be mitigated with thorough planning, setting performance goals, providing feedback, and mandating involvement/protected time.

Test preparation provides an additional opportunity for resident education. Whether it is for the ABSITE, FLS, or oral boards, preparatory courses can be of particular benefit to residents. Organization, critical feedback, and utilization of resources are keys to success. Resident feedback should be sought to further improve the course for future participants.

The newly arrived surgical interns provide a thirsty and captive audience for education. Intern orientation (i.e., "boot camps") is an excellent format for acclimating residents to what lies ahead and for teaching fundamental skills and procedures. Currently ACGME mandates resident preparedness for skills such as central line placement, intubation, and chest tube insertion. An interactive format with slides, handouts, hands-on training, and encouragement of questions is a general formula for success.

Indeed, almost any aspect of a surgeon's day can be an educational opportunity. The non-tangible aspects of surgery can arguably be learned only from "on-the-job" experiences and effective mentoring. These include conducting sensitive patient interviews, discussing medical errors, interacting with difficult patients, and "reading between the lines" in an effort to understand the patient's point of view and perception of understanding. An attending's quick summary of the dynamics of a difficult patient encounter can be invaluable to surgical residents. Furthermore, resident education on subjects such as public speaking, presentation skills, obtaining consent, and dictating operative reports can be very beneficial and generally is not associated with significant costs.

A final opportunity for resident education lies in mentoring. Prospective surgical residents are increasingly asking about mentorship programs during interviews. A surgeon mentor can help foster interests in research, subspecialties, innovation, or even surgical education. He or she can also help navigate residency – from selecting rotations and electives to counseling in areas of difficulty such as interpersonal relations, communication issues, difficult patients or patient outcomes, and medicolegal concerns. Career development coaching is an invaluable resource provided by mentors and guides the surgical resident in resume/CV building, interview preparation, job search strategies, networking, and transitioning to a new job.

Surgical Education of Residents: *Professional Aspects of Resident Education*

Surgical educators not only improve resident satisfaction and patient care; they also reap personal satisfaction, opportunities for research, avenues for career advancement, and potentially financial compensation. Faculty infrastructures vary but generally consist of a program director and one or more assistant program directors. These educational leaders organize and conduct didactic lectures and conferences, and other faculty members participate intermittently, particularly when their specialty fields are the topic of discussion. Compensation for this participation can be difficult to calculate, and anecdotally this is an area of research interest among academic leaders. It often consists of salary supplementation or relative value units (RVUs) applicable to a surgeon's productivity. These aspects are covered in Chap. 8. Moreover, such participation forms the basis of evaluation for one of the three academic pillars (education, research, and clinical performance). All educational efforts and experiences should be documented and feedback should be sought and collected in preparation for promotion and tenure review. Ultimately, the prospective surgeon educator should receive welcome guidance and instruction from the program director when pursuing educational opportunities.

Educational grants are often available from local and national academic societies as well as internally within academic institutions and can have tremendous positive implications for the aspiring surgeon educator. Educational grants from industry are also available; however, increasingly stringent conflict of interest policies at many institutions have limited this potential resource. Educational grants are described in more detail in Chap. 14.

For the surgeon educator who excels at the aforementioned endeavors and fully realizes their benefits, strong consideration should be given for further career advancement in the field of surgical education, such as the positions of Assistant Program Director or Program Director. This path begins with involvement in teaching opportunities; however, there are numerous other opportunities for faculty who are interested in increasing their involvement with the residency program. Such opportunities include active participation in the residency application process and individual mentoring of residents, especially those residents who may be struggling in the program. These contributions rarely go unnoticed and can often lead to a position as an Assistant Program Director. This position will introduce the faculty member to the inner workings and detailed requirements of running a residency. These faculty should also be encouraged to participate in educational conferences and organizations such as the Association of Program Directors in Surgery (APDS) and Association for Surgical Education (ASE). Within these groups are several open committees, faculty development workshops, and leadership courses that strengthen the curriculum vitae and candidacy of aspiring program directors. Further, surgical education research, a strong emphasis on mentoring, and broad networking among other surgical educators and residencies will better prepare one for the position of program director. While not mandatory, the majority of program directors are fellowship trained, perform clinical or basic science research, and have or have had grant funding. Guidance along this pathway can be provided by one's current program director, who is second to none in offering sound advice and will often happily accept an understudy to be groomed for their eventual replacement or to further propagate their success methods at another institution.

For those faculty interested in the regulatory and policy side of medical education, opportunities exist in Graduate Medical Education (GME) at programmatic, institutional, and national levels. Each institution and all of its programs must develop an educational curriculum that includes competency-based goals and objectives appropriate for each level of resident training. Programs must carefully document ongoing compliance with these educational goals as well as adherence to other ACGME mandated policies and procedures such as duty hours. This is an enormous and ever-increasingly complex task and involves resident and faculty performance evaluations, surveys and internal reviews, and formal ACGME site visits. Those interested in assisting in this process either for their own program or in participating in an internal review of another program within their institution are usually welcomed and should contact their program director and/or their institution's GME office to learn how to get involved. Additionally, the GME office of each institution is a valuable resource for faculty interested in education and typically offers many excellent faculty development workshops and seminars through the Academy of Medical Educators.

Surgical Education of Residents: *Summary*

The calling to teach in the field of surgery is felt by many, and benefits can be garnered by attendings, residents, and patients alike. The resourceful surgeon educator understands the intricacies of surgical residency (we have all been there) and can adapt to the myriad environments that the surgeon's career encompasses. By recognizing the educational opportunities that exist in all aspects of our work and adapting to the ever-increasing innovations that dominate the field, surgical residency will remain one of the most highly valued career training paths in our society.

Further Reading

Clarke R, Pugh C, Yates K, et al. The use of cognitive task analysis to improve instructional descriptions of procedures. J Surg Res. 2012;173(1):e37–42. Epub 2011 Oct 2.

Duggan P, Palmer E, Devitt P. Electronic voting to encourage interactive lectures: a randomized trial. BMC Med Educ. 2007;7:25.

Ko C, Escarce J, Baker L, et al. Predictors of surgery resident satisfaction with teaching by attendings. Ann Surg. 2005;241:373–80.

Pugh C, DaRosa D, Bell R. Residents' self-reported learning needs for intraoperative knowledge: are we missing the bar? Am J Surg. 2010;199:562–5.

Sanfey H, Cofer J, Hiatt J, et al. Service or education. Arch Surg. 2011;146:1389–95.

Schlitzkus L, Schenarts K, Schenarts P. Is your residency program ready for generation Y? J Surg Educ. 2010;67:108–11.

Vassiliou M, Feldman L, Andrew C, et al. A global assessment tool for evaluation of intraoperative laparoscopic skills. Am J Surg. 2005;190:107–33.

Chapter 4
Opportunities in Simulation Centers

Jacob R. Peschman and Jon C. Gould

Introduction

Simulation is rapidly becoming a vital component of any medical education process. As many medical and allied health professional schools move toward competency-based curriculums, objective measures of learning and structured curricula have become mandatory. Simulation is a highly efficient and effective means of learning that takes advantage of the experiential nature in which adults acquire new skills and judgment. Simulation is a partial solution for training multiple competencies simultaneously while in a controlled setting and assuring patient safety. Traditional training methods in medicine rely primarily on a didactic lecture format followed by performance of procedures by trainees on real patients. This aspect of the traditional training model introduces significant stresses and risks for both patients and the inexperienced trainees. Simulation allows us to bridge the gap between the classroom and the "real-life" experience. This is accomplished by challenging the trainee to make critical decisions and witness the results of those decisions in a controlled environment without risk to patient safety. Furthermore, simulation training supplies the educator with tools to create a limitless variety of scenarios for high-acuity, infrequently occurring clinical events. This gives trainees an opportunity to experience these events, wrestle with the difficulties involved, and do so at times that can be scheduled into a planned program, again without risk to human life.

Simulation-based learning always comes with an associated cost. If not in terms of actual dollars for simulation equipment or supplies, there is an opportunity cost and a time commitment for both instructors (who are often busy clinicians) and learners (in many cases learners are also care providers with many other responsibilities).

J.R. Peschman, MD • J.C. Gould, MD (✉)
Department of Surgery,
Medical College of Wisconsin,
Milwaukee, WI, USA
e-mail: jpeschma@mcw.edu; jgould@mcw.edu

C.M. Pugh, R.S. Sippel (eds.), *Success in Academic Surgery:*
Developing a Career in Surgical Education, Success in Academic Surgery,
DOI 10.1007/978-1-4471-4691-9_4, © Springer-Verlag London 2013

For these and other reasons, many institutions have invested in simulation centers. Space that is designed to facilitate simulation-based learning, dedicated staff to administer the education, shared resources (such as expensive high-fidelity manikins), and standardized curricula are just a few of the advantages of simulation centers and programs when compared to other learning and teaching modalities and venues.

The most recent requirements from the Accreditation Council for Graduate Medical Education (ACGME) effective July of 2012 continue to expand the role of simulation training for surgical residencies. Requirements for surgical residency programs have expanded from "Resources should include simulation and skills laboratories" to "Resources *must* include simulation and skills laboratories. These facilities must address acquisition and maintenance of skills with a competency-based method of evaluation." The American Board of Surgery now requires all surgeons to successfully pass the simulation-based Fundamentals of Laparoscopic Surgery (FLS) curriculum in order to become board eligible. This is likely the first step in what will ultimately become a larger requirement to demonstrate certain skills and competencies using simulation in order to attain certification or remain certified (Maintenance of Certification) to perform surgery. The opportunities for surgeons to get involved in simulation-based education and to push the field of high-stakes simulation-based assessment forward are numerous. Many of these opportunities exist in institutional simulation centers and programs. Clinicians providing care and training residents and students are in a unique position to recognize an educational need or training gap that might be effectively addressed using simulation. The most valuable and limited resource in many simulation centers is often the clinician who is willing and able to dedicate his/her time, energy, and enthusiasm to simulation-based education. Simulation centers are fertile grounds for enhancing one's education profile, conducting research, and embracing leadership opportunities.

What Is Simulation?

Simulation is a technique, not a technology. Simulation is the imitation or representation of one act or system by another. The overarching goal of simulation in healthcare education is enhanced efficiency, effectiveness, and patient safety. The purpose of a healthcare simulation may include any combination of one or more of the following: education, assessment, research, and/or health system integration.

Simulation can involve sophisticated high-tech equipment (e.g., a physiologic human manikin) or common inexpensive household materials (cutting a circle out of a piece of gauze as in the FLS curriculum). The complexity of the simulator is not necessarily directly related to its value as an educational tool. One must start with an educational goal or objective and work backward to define the best technology, equipment, or technique to accomplish this goal. There are many standardized educational curricula and simulation equipment available to use as educational aids. There are an innumerable educational needs and training gaps in healthcare, making simulation in surgical education ripe for innovation.

Why Simulation?

William Halsted is often cited as the founder of the current surgical training model. He implemented a system that involves graded learning and progressive responsibility for surgeon trainees in the 1890s. His intent was twofold. He wanted to make training among surgeons more uniform. Residency training would include basic science studies, typically 6 years of apprenticeship in the operating room under professors with a gradual increase in responsibility, and finally 2 years as a more autonomous "house surgeon." This model spread throughout the United States and became the basis for the modern surgical residency training system. A major advantage of Halsted's model (when it works well) is that the training can be tailored to the trainee. Contemporary pressures such as a focus on patient safety, resident work hour limitations, increasing demand for surgeons' and trainees' time outside of the OR (e.g., administrative responsibilities), and rapidly evolving techniques and technologies (i.e., laparoscopy or robotic surgery) have rendered this system impractical and insufficient. Our training and education system has evolved under these pressures. Much of the learning has necessarily and appropriately been moved out of the operating rooms and recently into simulation centers at many institutions.

Simulation Center Opportunities in Medical Student Education

Opportunities for surgeons to enhance the medical student core surgery rotation utilizing resources available in simulation centers are abundant. Many essential basic technical skills and tasks can be taught to medical students using simulation. Low-fidelity training models to teach intravenous catheter placement, basic suturing, knot tying, and abscess and/or fluid drainage (e.g., paracentesis or pleural effusion drainage) are readily available, inexpensive, and easy to use. Exposure to more sophisticated task trainers and simulators at an early stage of their education may actually foster an interest in surgery for students who may otherwise have been reluctant to consider this specialty as a career. A recent national trend has been to develop and offer elective simulation intensive courses for senior medical students interested in surgical specialties. The curricula for these so-called surgical boot camps vary between institutions. Common exercises include simulated pages and phone calls from nurses regarding patient care issues, training on the management of acute and potentially life-threatening situations using high-fidelity human patient manikins, and the early introduction to the FLS curriculum. Several recent studies have demonstrated the efficacy of these programs. It has been demonstrated that 4th-year medical students can successfully train on the FLS curriculum to preestablished proficiency levels equivalent to those of 5th-year surgical residents. This pre-training allows residency programs to invest valuable education time in more varied and advanced skills and task training earlier in the surgical residency. Other investigators have shown that senior medical students who complete competency-based preparatory courses are more confident surgical interns and perform at a higher level during their internship when compared to their peers who were not offered these pre-training opportunities. Considering the significant restrictions placed on first-year surgical resident's time under the current work hour reform rules and the multiple new responsibilities these young physicians are tasked with, the end of medical school may be the ideal time to develop the required basic skills and competencies. For this to be effective, a standardized curriculum offered to all medical students who match into a surgery residency would need to be offered at all medical schools.

Objective Structured Clinical Examinations (OSCEs) are becoming a common part of medical education training and evaluation for medical students. OSCEs are a core component of the United States Medical Licensing Examination (USMLE) Step 2 Clinical Skills (CS) exam required to obtain a medical license in the United States. Core competencies such as communication and professionalism which are important for all physicians can be developed, enhanced, and assessed through simulation. Medical students are an ideal subject group for many types of simulation-based research. By definition, medical students are often novices or naïve when it comes to exposure to particular surgical tasks or discrete surgical skills. This lack of prior exposure to many of these tasks is useful when it comes to investigating a new curriculum or simulator for preliminary evidence of construct validity (the ability to discriminate between users of different skill levels based on objective performance). When provided with access to simulators and simulation centers in the context of a validation study, medical students often prove to be enthusiastic and willing participants.

Opportunities in Simulation Centers with Surgical Resident Training and Education

In the current era of work hour limitations, public concerns regarding the relationship between patient safety and resident autonomy, increasing complexity of surgical procedures, and competition for cases between residents and postgraduate fellows, simulation is taking on an increasingly important role in residency training. Laparoscopic surgery was really the first discipline to take the learning for residents out of clinical practice (the operating room) and into the simulation lab. Laparoscopy lends itself well to simulation. An inexpensive box (video trainer) and recycled laparoscopic equipment are all that are needed to begin a simulation program in laparoscopic surgery. There are many "homegrown" curricula and laparoscopic skill tasks that have been described and utilized over the years. One curriculum in particular, the McGill Inanimate System for Training and Evaluation in Laparoscopic Skills (MISTELS), has been studied and evaluated extensively. Research involving medical students, surgical residents, and laparoscopic expert faculty has been conducted demonstrating that this curriculum is a valid tool for assessing and developing "real-world" laparoscopic surgical skill. This curriculum served as the basis for what has become the high-stakes curriculum known as the Fundamentals of Laparoscopic Surgery. The FLS curriculum has become a core component of most surgical residencies. Research has shown that training to preestablished proficiency levels on this curriculum results in improved performance in the operating room. These basic and generic non-procedural specific skills serve as the foundation for more advanced learning. In current practice, residents still do a fair amount of learning on patients in the operating room during clinical practice. There is currently no ideal substitute for learning how to operate on actual individual patients with unique anatomy and distinct technical challenges. Sophisticated virtual-reality laparoscopic simulators have been developed that allow trainees to perform entire simulated procedures (such as a virtual-reality cholecystectomy). These virtual-reality simulators tend to be extremely expensive without significant return on investment when compared to basic skills curricula such as FLS. Animal models are also often employed to teach residents and trainees surgery (e.g., the porcine model for laparoscopic cholecystectomy). Numerous opportunities exist for surgeons interested and willing to engage in these curricula and donate their time to teaching and mentoring young surgeons. Opportunities to advance the field of laparoscopic surgical simulation are numerous.

Laparoscopic technical skills are not the only kinds of manual skills that can or should be developed in the simulation lab. Procedures such as central line placement, chest tube placement, transesophageal echocardiography, and others can be successfully taught using inanimate models through simulation. Basic technical skills used in open surgery such as suturing, bowel anastomosis, and knot tying can be taught through simulation. Efforts are ongoing to develop more sophisticated simulators capable of teaching learners how to perform entire procedures such as inguinal hernia repair or Nissen fundoplication.

The technology to enable sophisticated virtual-reality surgical simulations exists and continues to evolve. Unfortunately, many of these training systems remain cost prohibitive. Significant work remains to develop inexpensive, validated, reliable, and high-stakes simulators to allow surgeons to deliberately develop and assess many of the technical skills required of practicing surgeons.

Opportunities in Simulation Centers with Practicing Surgeons

In the early 1990s, many practicing surgeons participated in short (1–3 day) courses before returning to their hospitals to begin performing laparoscopic cholecystectomy. Animal models of laparoscopic cholecystectomy were a part of the curriculum of many of these courses. Despite this fact, the first few years following the introduction of this new approach to a common operation were fraught with a significant increase in major biliary complications. With the evolution and advancement of simulation science and technology, surgeons' options for enhancing skills or developing new skills outside of a residency or fellowship training program are increasing. Animal models are still commonly employed when introducing surgeons to new technologies and procedures. Inanimate models and virtual-reality computer-based simulators are increasingly available. The fidelity and realism of these simulators continue to improve. Simulation centers offer ideal venues for surgeons to come learn the cognitive and technical skills inherent to new procedures they might wish to introduce into their surgical practices back home. Many of these courses can be structured to provide surgeons with continuing medical education credits. This provides additional incentive and motivation for surgeons to attend these courses. Many national surgical societies (such as the Society for American Gastrointestinal and Endoscopic Surgeons [SAGES] and the American College of Surgeons [ACS]) offer hands-on, simulation-based courses at their annual meetings. Often times, local simulation centers provide a more cost-effective and ideally suited venue for these courses.

The American Board of Surgery has recently moved away from recertification at 10-year intervals and toward ongoing Maintenance of Certification (MOC). Part 2 for the maintenance of certification is "lifelong learning and self-assessment." Surgeons can acquire CME credits which will count toward this requirement in simulation centers. Part 4 of maintenance of certification is "evaluation of performance in practice." This requirement is currently fulfilled by participating in quality assurance or outcomes databases. The American Board of Anesthesiology (ABA) currently allows board-certified anesthesiologists to meet part 4 MOCA (Maintenance of Certification in Anesthesiology) requirements by completing a MOCA-compliant simulation course. The ABA recognizes simulation training as an innovative approach to assess a physician's clinical and teamwork skills in managing critical events. It is likely that as high-stakes simulators and assessment tools develop, simulation and simulation centers will take on a more central role in the maintenance of certification process for surgeons as well.

Team Training

Simulation centers provide a perfect venue for providers who function as interdisciplinary teams in the clinical environment to enhance and develop their communication and teamwork skills. This kind of training is applicable to surgeons, non-surgeon physicians, and non-physicians (e.g., nurses and pharmacists) at all levels of training and experience (student, resident, and faculty). Crew resource management (CRM, sometimes also called crisis resource management) is a training method that has been employed for years in other industries, such as aviation, and is now making its way into healthcare team training. The overarching objective of CRM in healthcare is to improve patient safety. Providing safe healthcare depends on highly trained individuals with disparate roles and responsibilities acting together in the interest of the patient. Crew resource management in medicine is concerned not so much with the technical knowledge and skills required to perform specific operations or procedures but rather with cognitive and interpersonal skills needed to effectively manage a team-based, high-risk activity. Communication barriers across hierarchies, failure to acknowledge human fallibility, and a lack of situational awareness combine to cause poor teamwork that can lead to adverse events. TeamSTEPPS® is another teamwork system designed for healthcare professionals that is an evidence-based teamwork system designed to improve patient safety by improving communication and teamwork skills. TeamSTEPPS is based on more than 20 years of research and lessons learned from the application of teamwork principles. This training system was developed by the Department of Defense's Patient Safety Program in collaboration with the Agency for Healthcare Research and Quality (AHRQ). TeamSTEPPS materials are available for free on the AHRQ website. Simulation-based scenarios using the TeamSTEPPS process have been shown to result in improved teamwork. Many simulation centers include simulated operating rooms, high-fidelity human patient simulators, and sophisticated video equipment and technologies valuable for the post-simulation debrief. The debriefing is the critical teaching component of any high-fidelity, team training simulation session. The debriefing reveals patient care hazards, team strengths and weaknesses, and system issues that might not be immediately apparent otherwise. Team training has been shown to positively affect team-based behaviors, retention of personnel, and surgical outcomes.

Leadership Opportunities in Simulation Centers

The American College of Surgeons currently accredits simulation centers as Accredited Education Institutes (AEI). It is likely that this consortium of accredited simulation centers will play a central role in developing these curricula and administering any high-stakes simulation-based assessments required to maintain certification. The vision of the ACS AEI program is "To create a network of Education Institutes that offer practicing surgeons, surgical residents, medical students, and members of the surgical team the educational opportunities to address acquisition and maintenance of skills and to focus on new procedures and emerging technologies." To become a level I (comprehensive) AEI, institutions must meet certain standards for learners, curricula, resources, and technical support. An institutional commitment with dedicated staff and surgeon engagement is required. Opportunities to become involved in ACS-accredited simulation centers range from participation as a teacher, involvement as a curriculum champion, engagement in simulation research, and leadership positions in the simulation center. In addition to the position of Education Institute Director (25 % protected time), the Director of Surgical Program position also exists (10 % protected time) as a requirement to become ACS AEI certified. These positions are tremendous leadership opportunities that ambitious surgeons with an interest in surgical education can leverage to enhance their education and teaching portfolios.

Conclusions

The effectiveness of simulation as a teaching method and the value that simulation centers and programs can bring to the institution are readily apparent. Simulation centers and simulation-based training provide excellent opportunities for surgeons looking to advance their academic careers through teaching, education, and research.

Further Reading

Fried GM, Feldman LS, Vassiliou MC, Fraser SA, Stanbridge D, Ghitulescu G, et al. Proving the value of simulation in laparoscopic surgery. Ann Surg. 2004;240(3):518–25.

Gould JC. Building a laparoscopic skills lab: resources and support. JSLS. 2006;10(3):293–6.

Kim S, Ross B, Wright A, Wu M, Benedetti T, Leland F, et al. Halting the revolving door of faculty turnover: recruiting and retaining clinician educators in an academic medical simulation center. Simul Healthc. 2011;6(3):168–75.

Paige J. Surgical team training: promoting high reliability with nontechnical skills. Surg Clin North Am. 2010;90:569–81.

Chapter 5
Getting Involved at a National Level

Roger H. Kim

Introduction

Developing a successful career in surgical education is highly dependent on networking. Like so many other academic endeavors, success does not occur in a vacuum. For the junior faculty member just starting on his/her academic career, strong mentorship and engagement with like-minded personnel is critical. While there are a few institutions where education enjoys a robust support structure within the department of surgery, with multiple faculty members involved in educational endeavors, the vast majority of surgical educators do not enjoy such abundant availability of networking opportunities on a local level. Fortunately, there are many national professional organizations that provide the less fortunate among us with opportunities to engage in networking with other surgical educators.

A selection of the professional societies that are involved in surgical education is listed in Table 5.1. While this list is by no means comprehensive, it is representative of many of the key organizations that are heavily involved in education. In addition to this list, many surgical subspecialty organizations have forums or committees for education. These organizations provide additional opportunities for getting involved at a national level.

In this chapter, I will present some strategies for increasing one's involvement in surgical education at a national level, based primarily on my own personal experience. Some of the strategies described below may appear to be self-evident. However, I would assert that many of us were never instructed or advised on these matters during our surgical residencies. Most junior faculty, myself included, learned these lessons the hard and inefficient way – through personal experience, whether positive or negative. These reflections are presented here in order to allow

R.H. Kim, MD
Department of Surgery, Louisiana State University Health Sciences Center in Shreveport,
1501 Kings Hwy, 33932, Shreveport, LA 71130-3932, USA
e-mail: rkim@lsuhsc.edu

C.M. Pugh, R.S. Sippel (eds.), *Success in Academic Surgery:*
Developing a Career in Surgical Education, Success in Academic Surgery,
DOI 10.1007/978-1-4471-4691-9_5, © Springer-Verlag London 2013

Table 5.1 Professional societies important to surgical education

Society of University Surgeons (SUS)	www.susweb.org
Association for Academic Surgery (AAS)	www.aasurg.org
American College of Surgeons (ACS)	www.facs.org
Association for Surgical Education (ASE)	www.surgicaleducation.com
Association of Program Directors in Surgery (APDS)	www.apds.org
Association of American Medical Colleges (AAMC)	www.aamc.org
Surgical Council on Resident Education (SCORE)	www.surgicalcore.org
Accreditation Council for Graduate Medical Education (ACGME)	www.acgme.org
American Educational Research Association (AERA)	www.aera.net
American Medical Association (AMA)	www.ama-assn.org
National Board of Medical Examiners (NBME)	www.nbme.org
Association for Medical Education in Europe (AMEE)	www.amee.org

faculty to start their academic careers in the most efficient manner possible in regard to involvement on a national level. In addition, highlights of the opportunities at various national organizations will be outlined to serve as a resource guide.

Strategies for Increasing Involvement

As a preface to describing some strategies for increasing one's national profile, I would be remiss to not point out that junior faculty are often under two significant constraints: money and time. In this day and age of financial constraints, where surgical departments are often under significant budgetary pressures, the burden of annual membership dues and travel expenses associated with involvement in academic societies cannot be neglected. In addition, time spent away from home during such involvement can have a significant impact on one's clinical practice, academic endeavors, and personal life.

Because of this, each junior faculty needs to prioritize his/her involvement in organizations. This is often easier said than done. It can be tempting, especially early in one's career, to get involved in every organization and opportunity that presents itself. Resisting this temptation and selecting an appropriate distribution of time commitment will help prevent one from becoming spread too thin. As a general rule, depending on how much time and resources a faculty member has at his/her disposal, attendance at two or three national meetings per academic year may be a realistic goal, with membership in perhaps one or two additional organizations, including a state or regional surgical society. National organizations often have the advantage of presenting a greater opportunity for networking than local or regional societies, primarily due to their larger membership. However, smaller organizations at the local level can also be helpful to junior faculty, as they can offer opportunities that may not be easily accessible in larger societies at the early stages of one's career. The proximity of other members in state or regional societies can also make collaborative efforts easier than with members that are located in institutions on the other side of the country. The selection of which meetings to attend and which organizations to commit to is obviously a highly individualized decision and one that will depend on one's surgical subspecialty and career goals. Some of the opportunities at a few select organizations will be described later in this chapter.

Conduct at regional and national meetings can play a large influence on a junior faculty's trajectory for involvement. As with so many things in life, a happy medium is necessary. It is clearly not productive to be a social wallflower when it comes to these meetings. Getting one's name out there and on the mind of the leadership of a given organization is critical to opening the doors for involvement in that organization. Quietly attending a meeting and never speaking a word in a public forum would not be conducive to getting involved on a national level. Going up to the microphone after a research presentation to ask an insightful question or give a comment on a regular basis is helpful to increasing one's profile among an organization, especially if preceded by a concise introduction (name and current institution).

At the same time, a certain degree of restraint is needed. When commenting on another investigator's research in a public forum, doing so in a polite and complimentary manner is more effective than immediately launching into a scathing critique of the methodological flaws and limitations of the research. While going into "attack mode" may draw attention to oneself, it is not generally of the positive type and is unlikely to lead to opportunities to get involved in the organization, however correct the criticisms may be. This is an example of where emotional quotient (EQ) trumps intelligence quotient (IQ). It is far more productive to question and comment with a healthy dose of civility. Such professionalism does not go unnoticed by other members of a society, who are often in positions to help promote others to greater involvement.

Presenting at research meetings is another method of raising one's national profile. As more surgical societies recognize the importance of educational research, the opportunities for such presentations are becoming more abundant. Having one's name appear as an author on a regular basis in these research forums obviously has a significant impact in opening doors to greater involvement, whether as a moderator at future meetings or in terms of committee membership within the organization. These opportunities should be jumped on whenever possible. Performing assigned tasks in an exemplary fashion will lead to further advancement within the organization, as one's reputation continues to grow.

Finally, sharing credit and acknowledging achievement by others should be done as often as possible. By acknowledging the academic and clinical accomplishments by others in one's network of colleagues, these colleagues are more likely to reciprocate. Again, this is EQ at work. Sharing credit after a successful collaboration is not only a professional courtesy. This type of investment in human capital can also gain dividends in terms of reciprocation.

Opportunities for Involvement

The following sections are intended to highlight some of the opportunities for involvement in national organizations that are important to surgical education. These sections are not intended to provide a comprehensive list of every such opportunity. Clearly, such a list would be beyond the scope of this book. Instead, these selected examples from a handful of organizations are provided to serve as templates for opportunities that exist as other associations and societies.

Association for Academic Surgery

Founded in 1967, the Association for Academic Surgery (AAS) is focused primarily on research-based academic surgery and is geared towards junior faculty in the first 10 years of their academic career.

The Education Committee of the AAS has the mission of furthering the education of medical students, residents, and faculty in the field of surgery. Committee members are self-nominated and elected by a vote of the active membership to 2-year terms. One of the key tasks of the Education Committee is the planning of the annual Fundamentals of Surgical Research Course.

The AAS also has leadership positions for representatives to other societies dedicated to education – a representative to the ASE and a representative to the Association of American Medical Colleges (AAMC).

Jointly with the Society of University Surgeons (SUS), the AAS hosts the annual Academic Surgical Congress (ASC), the largest annual meeting of academic surgeons in the world. The profile of surgical education research at the ASC has steadily risen over the past decade, and the meeting now includes a dedicated Education Plenary Session to highlight the most compelling surgical education research reports. The official journal of the AAS is the *Journal of Surgical Research*, which publishes selected papers from the proceedings of the ASC, including manuscripts from education-based projects.

Society of University Surgeons

The Society of University Surgeons (SUS) was founded in 1938 and is one of the premier professional societies for academic surgery. One of the founding objectives of the SUS is the development of surgical resident training methods; thus, the SUS has surgical education as one of its core missions. Membership in the SUS is very selective and is based on four criteria: publications, grant funding, education/administrative activity, and participation in the ASC.

Among the standing committees of the SUS is the Committee on Surgical Education. Committee membership is by appointment by the president of the SUS and represents one of the prime opportunities for surgical educators to be involved on a national level.

As mentioned before, the SUS co-hosts the annual ASC with the AAS. The SUS is affiliated with the journal *Surgery*, which publishes many of the manuscripts that originate from presentations at the ASC, including many in educational research.

Table 5.2 Committees of the American College of Surgeons Division of Education

Advisory Committee on SESAP
Committee on Education
Committee on Continuous Professional Development
Committee on Resident Education
Committee on Medical Student Education
Committee on Allied Health Professionals
Committee on Emerging Surgical Technology and Education
Committee on Ethics
Committee for the Forum on Fundamental Surgical Problems
Committee on Video-Based Education
Program Committee
Patient Education Committee

American College of Surgeons

The American College of Surgeons (ACS) is the largest organization of surgeons in the world. The ACS Division of Education spearheads the organization's efforts in regard to education of practicing surgeons, residents, and medical students.

The ACS Division of Education conducts the annual Surgeons as Educators (SAE) course, which is a 6-day course offered each fall and is designed to enhance the abilities of surgeons as teachers and administrators of surgical education programs. Topics covered by the SAE course include teaching skills, curriculum development, educational administration and leadership, and performance/program evaluation. The SAE course is an excellent opportunity, not only for improving one's educational skill set, but also as a forum for networking with like-minded faculty from other institutions. The SAE course is discussed in greater detail in a later chapter of this book.

The ACS Division of Education has multiple committees available for involvement. Membership of all standing committees in the ACS is by election by the Board of Regents. The standing committees of the Division of Education are listed in Table 5.2.

Association for Surgical Education

The Association for Surgical Education (ASE) was founded in 1980 and represents institutions throughout the United States and Canada. The mission of the ASE is to promote, recognize, and reward excellence, innovation, and scholarship in surgical education. Membership in the ASE is open, and membership categories exist for residents and students. The ASE, in conjunction with the Association of Program Directors in Surgery (APDS) and the Association of Residency Coordinators in Surgery (ARCS), hosts the Surgical Education Week, an annual meeting held each spring, that is specifically geared towards providing a forum for individuals involved in surgical education.

Table 5.3 Standing committees of the Association for Surgical Education

Committee on Curriculum
Committee on Assessment and Evaluation
Committee on Faculty Development
Committee on Educational Research
Committee on Information Technology
Committee on Nurses in Surgical Education
Committee on Coordinators of Surgical Education
Committee on Clerkship Directors
Committee on Simulation
Committee on Graduate Surgical Education

The ASE is particularly well suited for junior faculty starting a career in surgical education due to its committee structure. Unlike other professional societies, the standing committees of the ASE are open to any member interested in getting involved. Committee meetings are generally held during the Surgical Education Week and during the American College of Surgeons Clinical Congress in the fall. The committees of the ASE are listed in Table 5.3.

The ASE also sponsors, through its foundation, the Surgical Education Research Fellowship (SERF). The SERF program is a 1-year, home-site fellowship designed to equip investigators to plan, implement, and report research studies in the field of surgical education. Accepted fellows are matched with a SERF advisor, who will serve as a mentor and consultant on the research project. Each SERF advisor is a respected and experienced researcher in surgical education. The SERF program has been highly successful and has jump-started the academic careers of many of the current leaders in surgical education research. More details on the SERF program are discussed in another chapter.

The official journal of the ASE is *The American Journal of Surgery*, which publishes selected papers from the Surgical Education Week.

Association of Program Directors in Surgery

The membership of the Association of Program Directors in Surgery (APDS) is comprised of the program directors and associate program directors of general surgical residency programs accredited by the Accreditation Council for Graduate Medical Education in the United States or by the Royal College of Physicians and Surgeons of Canada. Program directors and associate program directors automatically become members of the APDS upon their official designation as such. Other persons interested in graduate education in surgery are eligible for associate membership (non-voting). A resident membership category is also available.

As stated earlier, the APDS co-hosts the Surgical Education Week with the ASE and the ARCS. The official publication of the APDS is the *Journal of Surgical Education* (formerly titled *Current Surgery*), which dedicates one issue to the proceedings from the annual meeting.

Table 5.4 Committees of the Association of Program Directors in Surgery

Education/Mentorship Committee
Issues Committee
Ethics Committee
By-Laws Committee
Financial Committee
Curriculum Committee
Simulation Committee
Industry Committee

As with the other organizations mentioned, the APDS has several committees that provide opportunity for involvement. A current listing of these committees is provided in Table 5.4.

Association of American Medical Colleges

The Association of American Medical Colleges (AAMC) represents the 138 accredited US and 17 accredited Canadian medical schools, as well as almost 400 not-for-profit teaching hospitals and close to 100 academic societies. The AAMC supports professional development groups for leaders at its member institutions; membership in these groups requires appointment by the medical school dean in most cases. However, the Group on Educational Affairs (GEA) is open to any individual at a member medical school with a professional responsibility in education. The GEA hosts an annual Research in Medical Education Conference in conjunction with the annual meeting of the AAMC. The GEA also has annual meetings for each of its four designated AAMC regions: Southern, Central, Northeast, and Western. The national and regional meetings offer sessions and exhibits for research as well as teaching and learning opportunities. The AAMC and the GEA are not specifically intended for surgical educators exclusively; because of this, they offer opportunities for surgical educators to network with colleagues in other medical disciplines.

Academic Medicine is the official publication of the AAMC and is focused on issues involving undergraduate, graduate, and continuing medical education. *Academic Medicine* is currently ranked as the highest impact journal in the field of education in the scientific disciplines.

Conclusion

Multiple opportunities exist for getting involved at a national level in surgical education. There are a larger number of organizations that offer opportunities to network and collaborate with other like-minded faculty. A thoughtful and intentional strategy can aid in utilizing these opportunities to their maximal potential to increase one's national profile.

Further Reading

Capella J, Kasten SJ, Steinemann S, Torbeck L, editors. Guide for researchers in surgical education. Woodbury: Cine-Med Publishing; 2010.

Carnegie D. How to win friends and influence people. New York: Simon and Schuster; 1981.

Goleman D. Emotional intelligence: 10th anniversary edition: why it can matter more than IQ. New York: Bantam; 2006.

Chapter 6
Getting Promoted as a Surgical Educator

Meghana Vellanki, Gregory T. Horn, and Steven B. Goldin

Introduction

Prior to accepting a job as an assistant professor, one should have defined both their short-term (5 years) and long-term (10 years) career goals. Success as a faculty member can be measured using various metrics, but for the purposes of this chapter, promotion to associate and then full professor will be the yardstick. Reaching these milestones requires careful planning and institutional support, which should be included in any employment contract.

Several academic surgical career pathways exist for faculty to achieve promotion. Historically, academic surgeons oversaw a basic science laboratory, taught residents and medical students, and had a specialized clinical practice. The majority of a faculty person's time was spent doing research, speaking, publishing manuscripts, and obtaining funding from outside sources. Today, it is rare for surgeons to follow this "clinical investigator" pathway as it requires most of a faculty person's time to be spent doing research. It is now more common to see academic surgeons following a "clinical educator" or "clinical researcher" pathway for career advancement. The basic career pathways are shown in Fig. 6.1. This shift away from the clinical investigator pathway has largely been related to the difficulty many institutions have in supporting full-time clinical investigators which require tremendous

M. Vellanki, BS
Department of Medicine, University of South Florida,
Morsani College of Medicine, Windermere, FL, USA

G.T. Horn, BA
Department of Surgery, University of South Florida,
Morsani College of Medicine, Tampa, FL, USA

S.B. Goldin, MD, PhD (✉)
Department of Surgery, University of South Florida,
Tampa General Hospital, Tampa, FL, USA
e-mail: sgoldin@health.usf.edu

C.M. Pugh, R.S. Sippel (eds.), *Success in Academic Surgery:*
Developing a Career in Surgical Education, Success in Academic Surgery,
DOI 10.1007/978-1-4471-4691-9_6, © Springer-Verlag London 2013

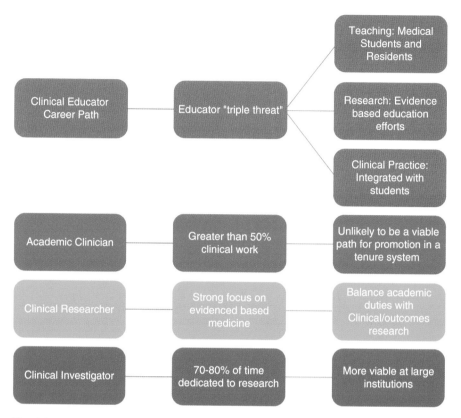

Fig. 6.1 Pathways for promotion

resources and dedicated time. The clinician investigator pathway is, however, still a viable route to promotion at some of larger institutions with significant resources. Depending upon the institution, the clinical investigator pathway may also be the only viable pathway available to achieve tenure status. The importance of tenure, however, should also be discussed. Although tenure at many institutions still guarantees academic freedom, it does not guarantee income or continued progress within the institution. Thus, although tenure may be considered an incentive, the real goal of most faculty members should be promotion and career advancement. Understanding the promotion and tenure process at your individual institution is important, and understanding how tenure fits into one's career goals often depends upon the chosen career pathway.

University and departmental financial needs have now resulted in surgeons at many institutions choosing either the clinical educator or clinical researcher pathways for promotion. Most surgeons cannot spend 75 % of their time as a clinical investigator dedicated to research as is required upon receipt of many NIH-funded grants. Therefore, these alternative pathways for career advancement and promotion are gaining more widespread acceptance within many institutions that wish to keep productive and valuable faculty members. The alternative pathways for career advancement include the clinical educator, clinical researcher, and academic clinician pathways. The academic clinician pathway may be an option at some institutions, but overall is not a viable pathway for promotion at most institutions and is often the pathway taken by those accepting positions without clearly defined goals and clinical responsibilities.

The importance of educational endeavors was poorly defined in the past. Education, however, has now become a central component of the mission of most academic medical centers. In 1999, Sachdeva et al. suggested that an "educator's pyramid" be incorporated into every department as a means to offer recognition and awards to the faculty based on a broad definition of educational scholarship [1]. Recent recommendations from the American Surgical Association's Blue Ribbon Committee on Surgical Education support this concept and recommend increasing the focus on educational scholarship including selecting faculty working on the educational mission. This chapter details how a surgeon may follow the clinical educator pathway for promotion and career advancement.

Accepting Your First Job

Short- and long-term career goals should be defined prior to accepting a job. This is one key to success. Knowing one's career goals is important for negotiating an employment contract. Unfortunately, most physicians are inexperienced in negotiating and may make mistakes that go unrecognized until much later. When exploring potential positions, both the individual physician and the institutional goals should be compared. It is important to ensure that the institution can provide the required support and that they are committed also to the success of the relationship. The institutional commitment may sometimes be apparent by the current level of support it provides to a program already in existence. For example, if your career goals include significant outcomes research, are there other successful surgeons present at that institution working in a large funded outcomes group or does the group not exist? Developing a program from scratch without mentoring is a recipe for failure at any institution including those with good intentions. The same analogy can be made for those interested in following a clinical educator pathway. Does the institution support salaries for educational work? Is there an educational research group at the institution? Does the department have a surgical educator? Does the chairman of surgery support education? Understanding the level of commitment of the institution and the department is one key component to being successful.

Individual support can be provided in several forms. Departments may provide advanced training, mentoring, protected time, and financial assistance. Institutions stressing high volumes of clinical activity may leave one without time for scholarly research or adequate time to develop the educational programs needed for career advancement. Faculty excitement for a clinically busy position should be tempered by the requirements for long-term success [2, 3]. Most academic positions presume it will take approximately 5 years for promotion from assistant professor to associate professor and another 5 years to reach the level of professor. Most good educational programs that incorporate scholarly activity (research) take at least 1–2 years to develop with the publication process taking even longer. Do not let a busy clinical practice become an excuse for the lack of scholarly activity, since most Promotions and Tenure Committees will be looking for scholarly activity as well as teaching performance. Become familiar with the institutions' promotion and tenure processes, guidelines, and requirements since they do differ between institutions.

Mentoring

Mentors are important for the success of all young faculty. Each faculty member may have multiple mentors including those from medical school and residency. Mentors can offer great advice when it comes to accepting a first position. One may have a mentor for each area of interest. For example, one might choose a mentor for difficult cases (clinical mentor) and a mentor for educational research (research mentor). The mentor may or may not be at the same institution, as long as they are available and willing to assist or advise. A key aspect of any mentor is that they are senior enough to have their mentee's best interest at heart. The perfect mentor has time to devote to his mentee and his mentee's career goals. They do not usually need to advance their own careers at the mentee's expense. Mentors should be friends, offer opportunities and sometimes resources, advise regarding promotion and employment, and have intricate knowledge of the processes. A really good mentor is very valuable and not always easy to find.

Leadership Positions and Administrative Appointments

Success as a clinical educator, by definition, requires one to have an important role as an educator. Simply giving a lecture or instructing or teaching medical students or residents in the clinic or operating room is not enough to be defined as a clinical educator and is more consistent with that of an academic clinician. Leadership positions for clinical educators include the clerkship director for the medical students, program director for the residents, and the vice chairman of surgical education. The assistant clerkship director and assistant program director roles can also be helpful, but do not have the same level of involvement or responsibility that belongs to the actual director. These assistant positions, however, may be stepping stones to the actual director position. The directors usually participate on a variety of institutional committees. The director title may also help one obtain leadership positions in various national organizations. The title, if backed by authority, also simplifies the implementation of curriculum changes and various research projects aimed at educational topics which will be keys to scholarly productivity and overall success.

The clerkship director role is probably also preferable to that of the program director at most institutions. Most surgeons may feel that the program director position is more desirable for career advancement, but this is probably not the case. Although program directors play an integral role in the functioning of the department and the residency program, most medical schools exist for medical students and most state aid is directed towards undergraduate education. The clerkship director is also better entwined within the hierarchy of the medical school, which is probably why clerkship directors have higher promotion rates than their peers.

Teaching

Clerkship directors, program directors, and faculty all need to teach. Good teachers must also be good clinicians. Surgeons that teach a lot are usually recognized for their efforts within the institution. Although some may view teaching as a burden that slows patient flow and clinical productivity, it may actually help physicians build their practice as word of mouth spreads about their abilities and interests within the institution. Teaching can help new faculty members build their practices and a "reasonable practice" is expected for promotion at most institutions.

Clinical educators must teach extensively and must also teach well. There are a variety of courses, web-based materials, and seminars available to assist faculty in improving their teaching abilities. Some courses are given as breakout sessions at national organizational meetings like the Association of Academic Surgery (AAS) or the Association for Surgical Education (ASE). The American College of Surgeons (ACS) offers a yearly course called the Surgeons as Educators course. The AAS offers a course on research called "The Fundamentals of Surgical Research" that contains a section on educational research. The ASE offers a yearly course for clerkship directors and coordinators on running the surgical clerkship, and the Association of Program Directors in Surgery (APDS) offers a course for all new surgery program directors. Clinical educators should consider negotiating these courses into their employment contract or include them in discussions when asked to assume the role of an educational director.

Second, many organizations have formal methods in place for measuring teaching proficiency, quality, and quantity. This, however, may not be true of your institution, and if your institution does not do this, a teaching portfolio is mandatory. All faculty, regardless of their career track, should carefully document "all" of their teaching activities. At institutions that do document teaching, it may only be certain aspects of teaching that are recorded and many teaching events may go undocumented. An example is seen when medical schools document lectures given to the undergraduates. Medical student lectures may have a paper trail, but lectures given to residents or the community as CME activities may go undocumented. Teaching portfolios are good ways to ensure credit is received for all types of teaching activities which are important considerations for most Promotion and Tenure Committees.

Table 6.1 Components of a teaching portfolio

1. Reflective statement	A one-page statement about your teaching philosophy
2. Introductory statement	Describe yourself, your teaching responsibilities, and percent effort devoted to teaching
3. Important contributions as an educator	This critical section should be updated with your accomplishments frequently. This section includes:
	A. Direct teaching activities
	B. Curriculum and material development
	C. Learner assessment
	D. Educational scholarship/creation of enduring educational materials
	E. Educational administration and leadership
	F. Professional development in education
	G. Mentorship and guidance
4. Appendix	Include supporting documents for Sect. 6.3 and list awards and honors

Teaching Portfolio

Teaching portfolios are becoming significantly more important for those in the clinical educator pathway. Teaching portfolios should be kept and maintained like a curriculum vitae. Teaching portfolios showcase accomplishments, document scholarly activity and teaching, and assist one at the time of promotion. Various methods of organizing a teaching portfolio exist and there may be a specific format used by your institution. The Association for Surgical Education recommends that the portfolio be arranged around four key areas listed in Table 6.1. A sample teaching portfolio can be downloaded at the ASE Educational Clearing House website http://www.surgicaleducation.com/educational-clearinghouse which also contains a large number of other good teaching materials and resources.

Medical School Committees

Participation in medical school committees is very important for career progression. There are several committees that directly involve education and these committees may have various names at different institutions. These committees include the Clerkship Directors Committee, Curriculum Committee, Academic Performance Review Committee, and Admissions Committee. There may also be other committees that are institutionally relevant. Perhaps there is a committee on educational research or committees that deal with scholarly concentrations that may be relevant to education.

Table 6.2 Organizations offering educational resources [4]

Alliance for Clinical Education	http://www.allianceforclinicaleducation.org
American College of Surgeons	http://www.facs.org
Association for Academic Surgery	http://www.aasurg.org
Association for Surgical Education	http://www.surgicaleducation.com
Association for Medical Education in Europe	http://www.amee.org
Association of American Medical Colleges	http://www.aamc.org
Association of Program Directors in Surgery	http://www.apds.org/index.htm
Society of University Surgeons	http://www.susweb.org

Committee involvement by the clerkship director keeps them up to date and informed about things happening in the medical school. Involvement on the committees also enables the participant to get to know those of influence within the medical school who will be important for promotion. Committee participation is essential, but participation on every committee is not. Participation on the Clerkship Directors, Curriculum, and Academic Performance Committees improves a clerkship director's ability to perform their job. Residency program directors have much less opportunity to interact in this manner and many of the committees that are important for clerkship directors have nothing to do with managing the residency. Thus, committee involvement is often a better fit for clerkship directors than program directors. Program directors, however, can participate on undergraduate educational committees including the Admissions Committee as well as the graduate medical education committee within the hospital. Most committees will have various retreats and working subcommittees. Chairing a subcommittee or the actual committee is an opportunity to demonstrate leadership among peers, builds an internal reputation, and demonstrates value to the institution. The reputation one develops is important for success.

Professional Societies and Committees

Professional societies provide for excellent venues to pursue educational endeavors. Table 6.2 contains some of the professional organizations that are either centered around education or have major areas focused on education.

Promotion at most institutions is based upon feedback received by outside reviewers. At the time of promotion, faculty submit the names of outside reviewers to the Promotion and Tenure Committee. Promotion, therefore, requires development of a national reputation which can be accomplished by involvement in these organizations. Several of these organizations are aimed at young faculty and/or have committees that encourage junior faculty member participation. The AAS is one of these organizations and has a yearly meeting with the Society of University Surgeons (SUS). This meeting has sections devoted entirely to educational research.

A clerkship or program director title can be helpful when running for election for these committees. These titles clearly demonstrate a commitment to education and the profession. Participation in the AAS, via committee involvement, is one requirement for selection into the SUS which can also be helpful for career advancement. Another organization that should be joined is the Association for Surgical Education (ASE). They have a yearly meeting with the Association of Program Directors in Surgery (APDS). The ASE has an open-door policy for committee members and you become a member of their committees by simply showing up to the committee meetings. Most organizational committees meet at their own annual meeting and at the American College of Surgeons meeting. They may also have other meetings during the year. By participation in these committees and their working groups, one can become chair of a committee and get to know colleagues from throughout the country. The people you meet will eventually write your letters for promotion.

Research

Promotion does require publication. The increasing clinical demands experienced by faculty at many institutions can make publishing and doing research difficult. Clinical investigators with NIH funding usually spend at least 75 % of their time doing research as a requirement of grant acquisition. Those following a clinical educator pathway cannot spend 75 % of their time doing research activities. In fact, it is suggested that clerkship directors be given approximately 50 % protected time to ensure that their educational mission is carried out properly. In reality, however, most clerkship directors do not have this luxury of 50 % protected time and need to maintain a busy clinical practice and the quality of the clerkships they are responsible for overseeing. Having a good assistant or surgical clerkship coordinator really helps offset some of the workload and is really a requirement if one accepts the job as a director.

Everyone is familiar with the framework of evidence-based medicine. Faculty involved with education should be working in the framework of "evidence-based teaching." Evidence-based teaching means that educators should use teaching methods which have demonstrated superiority over other methods in teaching. Defining these methods and other issues directly related to learners is what defines educational research.

All research has a time commitment, and those working in a clinical educator pathway have multiple responsibilities. As mentioned, a clerkship coordinator can really help reduce some of the workload. This can help to free some time for research. For those following a clinical educator pathway, research should be combined with daily activities to improve time management and efficiency. Directing a clerkship, course, or residency program has advantages which should be utilized, which include a constant supply of learners, routine and frequent data collection, and routine measurement of proficiencies. Asking learners questions and collecting data is done for every course. Making the questions scholarly involves a careful literature review, obtaining IRB approval, collecting data, and publishing results. This final product or manuscript is another key for promotion. Educational research can also be presented at multiple forums. The AAS, ASE, and American College of Surgeons (ACS) meetings have sections devoted entirely to educational research. Other meetings like the Association of American Medical Colleges (AAMC) are also good forums for presenting educational research. Many journals including surgical journals are also publishing educational research papers. Presenting at national meetings is another way to build a reputation in the field and gain outside respect.

This chapter is not designed to discuss educational research; however, the need for training and funding are two educational topics that deserve brief mention because they relate to promotion. The process of actually doing educational research was overly simplified above. It is important to realize that doing educational research properly requires mentorship and training. Junior faculty entering a clinical educator pathway should have at least one mentor for educational research. Although it is possible to start an educational research program from scratch, working with others at your institution or other institutions may result in the best and most productive outcomes.

There are no shortcuts for learning how to do good educational research. Towards this end, a variety of training programs are available which teach one how to do educational research properly. These programs are highly recommended for anyone interested in really understanding how to design studies, collect and process data, analyze data, produce publishable manuscripts, and compete for funding. These programs include master's programs in education or public health, course work in biostatistics and epidemiology, and structured research programs like the Surgical Education Research Fellowship (SERF) program sponsored by the ASE. The SERF program is probably unique in that it matches individuals with an educational research mentor. Table 6.3 lists some of the options available for those interested in additional training in education and educational research. Completing one of these programs will also help to enhance your portfolio.

Educational research funding is difficult to obtain. Most educational research, however, can be done using a very small budget coupled to the facilities and resources that are already in place for teaching. Funding, however, can be sought from several surgical organizations including the AAS and the ASE. Large device manufacturing corporations and pharmaceutical companies may also be willing to fund some educational research projects. Internal organizational grants can also sometimes be obtained especially if they involve topics with clear educational value for their learners. Although obtaining outside funding for educational research projects is difficult, it is considered significant by Promotion and Tenure Committees.

Table 6.3 Opportunities for professional development [4]

School of public health	A school of public health is a great resource for classes teaching how to conduct research. An MPH degree with certification in biostatistics, epidemiology, and research methods is available
Master's program in education	A master's program in education to improve skills in communication and education
ACS Surgeons as Educators Course	A 1-week course offered by the American College of Surgeons
University of Illinois at Chicago Masters in Health Professions Education Program	Courses on management, leadership, scholarship, curriculum, assessment, program evaluation, primary care education, clinical decision making, medical humanities, and ethics. Coursework can be completed on campus or online
Association for Surgical Education Surgical Education Research Fellowship (SERF)	A 1-year fellowship designed to provide participants with the skills and knowledge needed to complete research in surgical education. This fellowship is done at one's own institution
University of California, Los Angeles Medical Education Fellowship	A 2-year program that includes curriculum development, educational leadership, scholarly endeavors, and teaching skills
Harvard Macy Institute	Health-care education programs that teach participants methods for translating their knowledge and capabilities into organization-wide improvements

Clinical Experience and Balancing an Academic Career

A successful career as an academic surgeon requires a careful balancing act between patient care, educational research, leadership and administrative positions, and teaching. Juggling these roles requires a significant time commitment and dedication. Organization and efficiency is fundamental to maintaining a busy schedule that allows one to achieve optimal clinical and academic productivity.

A fundamental trait of a good academic surgical teacher is clinical expertise. To receive respect in the department and the institution, one must have a good clinical practice and be an expert surgeon. Thus, developing a solid practice is important. At the same time, approximately 25–50 % of one's time will need to be dedicated to leadership positions, administrative duties, mentoring, research, and pursuing educational efforts. These factors are all considered important for those in the clinical educator pathway for promotion. Due to the transformations taking place in academic surgery, it is critical to establish each of these roles as a clinician educator.

Historically, clinical educators have not had protected time like the traditional clinician investigator. This is now changing and some institutions provide significant financial support for their educators, which helps to offset clinical productivity expectations. One should determine this level of support prior to accepting a position

Fig. 6.2 Flowchart showing the components for a physician following the surgical educator pathway

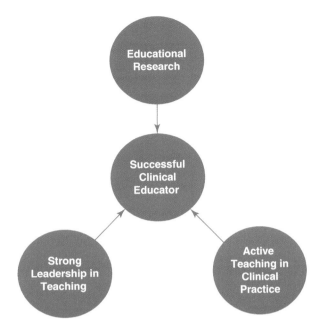

because it is different at each institution. Those with more support can spend more time teaching and in research activities. As mentioned, those that focus mainly on clinical responsibilities or follow an academic clinician pathway are less likely to be promoted so a clear balance between clinical responsibilities, teaching, and research is essential to ones' success.

Conclusions

The clinical educator pathway is a viable pathway for promotion at most institutions. Careful planning is required to successfully negotiate this and any promotional pathway. The true triple threat of being a busy clinician, having a research laboratory with NIH funding, and being a great teacher is truly rare. The opportunity for one to be this type of triple threat (Fig. 6.2), however, may exist in the clinical educator pathway if one develops a clinical practice, takes leadership positions with respect to teaching at both the institutional and national levels, and develops a successful educational research program. Following this roadmap as a clinical educator should result in a fulfilling successful academic surgical career.

References

1. Sachdeva AK, Cohen R, Dayton MT, et al. A new model for recognizing and rewarding the educational accomplishments of surgery faculty. Acad Med. Dec 1999;74(12):1278–87.

2. Staveley-O'Carroll K, Pan M, Meier A, Han D, McFadden D, Souba W. Developing the young academic surgeon. J Surg Res. Oct 2005;128(2):238–42.
3. Buckley LM, Sanders K, Shih M, Hampton CL. Attitudes of clinical faculty about career progress, career success and recognition, and commitment to academic medicine. Results of a survey. Arch Intern Med. 2000;160(17):2625–9.
4. Sanfey H, Gantt NL. Career development resource: academic career in surgical education. Am J Surg. Jul 2012;204(1):126–9.

Chapter 7
Leadership Courses

Amalia Cochran

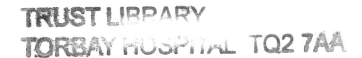

Organization-Led Courses

Programs in physician leadership development are sponsored by a number of national organizations. While some of these are general in scope, others specifically target women and minorities. In addition, surgeon-specific programs have been developed by the American College of Surgeons, the Association for Academic Surgery, and the American Society of Transplant Surgeons. These courses are summarized in Table 7.1.

Physician Leadership Development

The American College of Physician Executives (ACPE) focuses on leadership and management skills for physicians with the goal of having more physicians in medical executive roles. The ACPE offers training via distance learning, live conferences offered throughout the year at various venues, or a customized leadership development program with on-site training. ACPE has a particular focus on the business side of medicine, with an emphasis on issues of healthcare policy, management, and delivery.

Female and minority faculty in medicine and sciences are the target audience for the programs that have been developed by the American Association of Medical Colleges (AAMC). The Group on Women in Medicine and Science within the AAMC hosts an Early Career Women Faculty Professional Development Seminar each summer and a Mid-Career Women Faculty Professional Development Seminar

A. Cochran, MD
Department of Surgery, University of Utah,
Salt Lake City, UT, USA
e-mail: amalia.cochran@hsc.utah.edu

C.M. Pugh, R.S. Sippel (eds.), *Success in Academic Surgery:*
Developing a Career in Surgical Education, Success in Academic Surgery,
DOI 10.1007/978-1-4471-4691-9_7, © Springer-Verlag London 2013

Table 7.1 Organization-led courses

Organization	Target audience	Duration
American College of Physician Executives	Physician executives	3–5 days (live courses)
AAMC Early Career	Women	4 days
	Assistant professors	
AAMC Mid-Career	Women	4 days
	Associate professors	
AAMC Minority Faculty	Underrepresented groups	4 days
	Assistant professors	
ELAM	Senior women faculty	1 year
ACS Surgeons as Leaders	Surgeons, all practices types	3 days
ACS Residents as Teachers and Leaders	Mid-level and senior surgical residents	2 days
AAS Career Development Course	Senior residents	1 day
	Fellows	
	Junior faculty	
	Surgeons	
ASTS/Kellogg Leadership Development Program	Clinical transplant surgeons	4 days
	Administrative transplant program leaders	

each fall. The Early Career seminar is designed for assistant professors and strives to provide them with strategies for career building in academic medicine. Key objectives include creating a structure for achieving leadership goals, networking, and identifying skill areas in need of development. The Mid-Career seminar addresses issues primarily relevant to those at the associate professor level. Skills emphasized in this seminar are those related to formation and use of teams, with a particular emphasis on effective collaboration. Leadership topics in the Mid-Career seminar include communication skills, institutional finance, and management issues.

The AAMC also hosts an annual Minority Faculty Development Seminar for junior faculty who are members of underrepresented racial and ethnic minority groups. This seminar assists participants in identifying their professional development goals and establishing a pathway to pursue these goals. A significant focus of the seminar is the navigation of the retention, promotion, and tenure process in academic medicine. Networking, grant writing, and communications are also emphasized.

The Drexel University Executive Leadership in Academic Medicine (ELAM) program spans 1 year and is the only national program for senior women faculty at schools of medicine, public health, and dentistry. The program includes executive education, leadership assessments and coaching, and networking and mentoring activities for participants. ELAM has over 700 graduates who serve in diverse leadership positions both nationally and internationally. ELAM is the leadership program that has the most outcome data to demonstrate the leadership development value of participation.

Surgeon-Specific Programs

The American College of Surgeons (ACS) Surgeons as Leaders course is designed for both academic and community surgeons. This 3-day course addresses leadership at all levels of an organization and helps surgeons to acquire essential skills; the course's purpose explicitly excludes management of people, groups, and organizations. The five major blocks of content include the following topic areas: attributes of a leader, aligning values and leading change, building and maintaining team effectiveness, leading oneself, and the art and principles of leadership. Faculty and planners for this course include nationally and internationally recognized surgical leaders.

The ACS has recently developed a course entitled Residents as Teachers and Leaders. Nonclinical skills like teaching and leadership often go neglected in residency program curricula; this weekend-long course provides a method to remedy those practice gaps. The course is designed for mid- and senior-level surgical residents and endeavors to give them the tools to become more effective leaders for their teams and within their institutions. This is the only current opportunity that is explicitly designed for and delivered to surgeons in training.

The Association for Academic Surgery (AAS) Fall Career Development Course includes information on planning and development in an academic career as well as capitalizing on committee involvement locally and nationally. An additional focus of this program is the development of a research program, including acquisition of extramural funding. This course is delivered in tandem with the AAS Fundamentals of Research Course, providing a 2-day intensive workshop for senior residents embarking upon an academic career or junior faculty trying to get a strong start in academic surgery and in surgical leadership.

The American Society of Transplant Surgeons (ASTS) collaborates with the Kellogg School of Management for their transplantation-specific leadership development program, which is designed for both clinical and administrative leaders of transplant centers. The distinctive demands of leading a transplant program, particularly with the need for collaboration within and between institutions as well as the unique regulatory environment, generate singular needs in transplant surgeons and program administrators. Therefore, this program has a heavy focus on the business and regulatory aspects of leading a transplant program as well as including sessions on fundamental leadership skills such as team building, collaboration, and strategic analysis.

Institution-Based Courses

Leadership programs created by academic institutions are often executive programs, allowing participants to travel to those institutions for a focused period of time to acquire additional knowledge and training. While many of these programs are designed for specialized development in healthcare leadership and policy, some are neither physician specific nor healthcare specific. Programs of this more comprehensive nature place the onus on the attendee to independently identify those areas in which they would benefit from additional training and then to select a program best suited to their needs.

Institutional Courses with National and International Attendance Pools

A number of nationally prominent institutions sponsor executive education programs. Some of these programs are designed like many of the organization-led programs, with their programming conducted in an intensive workshop for 3 or 4 days. Others require participants to travel to their site a few times a year for a more in-depth "immersion" experience.

The Harvard Business School (HBS) Healthcare Initiative integrates healthcare research, educational program, and collaboration. The overall goal of this program is to develop leaders who work to provide best care in a cost-efficient manner. To that end, they have a traditional MBA program with the ability to design a narrower concentration area within healthcare delivery. HBS also has an extensive executive education program that has both comprehensive immersion-style courses in general management and leadership development as well as shorter healthcare-specific courses. HBS does offer a comprehensive 9-month course in managing healthcare delivery that entails 3 weeks of on-site coursework with projects required between modules.

Also at Harvard, the Harvard Macy Institute provides professional development for educational leaders in the healthcare professions. The Harvard Macy program has the goal of helping participants to develop the skill sets to lead organizational change in medical education as well as to drive innovation. Their "Educators in Healthcare Professions" and "Program for Leading Innovations in Healthcare and Education" use an executive education, short-term residential format to train medical educators as leaders; the Harvard Macy Institute is currently unique in its integration of medical education, business practices, education theory, and innovation.

The Stanford Graduate School of Business hosts a number of executive education programs in both personal and organizational leadership, though none are explicitly designed for healthcare. The Stanford Executive Program is a 6-week intensive course offering a general management curriculum; some form of this course has been offered for 60 years, and it was described by the institution as their "flagship" executive education program. Organizational leadership courses include "Leading Change and Organizational Renewal" and "Managing Talent for Strategic Advantage." Personal leadership courses focus on individual-level skills and include specific leadership programs for Asian-American executives and for women leaders.

Brandeis University hosts a 6-day surgeon-focused leadership course in health policy and management through the Heller School for Social Policy and Management. This course is cosponsored by the American College of Surgeons, the Thoracic Surgery Foundation for Research and Education, and 14 other surgical societies. Thirty to thirty-five physician leaders attend annually. This course specifically addresses the business of healthcare delivery, the process of healthcare policy and reform, and techniques for team leadership and conflict resolution.

The Center for Creative Leadership (CCL) is a nonprofit, multicampus educational institution with a global emphasis on using executive education programs to further leadership education and research. CCL offers core programs for individuals at all stages of their leadership trek, from leadership fundamentals for the new leader to leadership "at the peak," with interval steps between these two points. Specialized skill development may occur through working programs that target particular interests or needs of learners, with these courses lasting from 3 to 5 days. CCL also has the distinction of using program evaluation exercises to generate peer-reviewed publications and white papers.

Institutional Courses of Regional Interest

Many regional institutions host executive or professional educational programs, some culminating with the award of an MBA. Few of these are healthcare specific. Examples of broad-based regional programs include the University of Wisconsin Executive Education Course in Leadership Beyond Management, a 5-day course emphasizing the acquisition of leadership skills by individuals in managerial roles. The Duke Leadership Program at the Fuqua School of Business provides a similar undifferentiated option in leadership training. This 5-day course is promoted to anyone with "current or anticipated leadership responsibilities." Programs with comparable content and of like duration are available at business schools across the United States.

The University of Utah has a unique "Leadership Development for Healthcare Professionals" executive education course for healthcare providers and administrators who seek to improve their leadership and managerial skills. This course has 1 week of intensive coursework that is followed by five 2-day modules. The program uses real-life healthcare cases to reinforce key business practices using a multidisciplinary approach.

Conclusion

Surgeons with an interest in developing their leadership skills have diverse resources available to do so. The courses available for different career stages and interests provide broad opportunities for learners to have their individual needs met. Although these resources are associated with financial and time costs for busy clinicians, development of leadership skills for all surgeons benefits our patients, our practices, and our work environments.

Further Reading

Browning HW, Torain DJ, Patterson TE. Collaborative healthcare leadership: a six-part model for adapting and thriving during a time of transformative change. Center for Creative Leadership White Papers. 2011. http://www.ccl.org/leadership/pdf/research/CollaborativeHealthcareLeadership.pdf. Accessed 15 July 2012.

Campos HC, Friedman SR, Haddad AE, Campos F, Morahan PS. Chapter 14. Evaluation of health professions leadership and management and programs that teach these competencies. In: McGaghie WC, editor. International best practices for evaluation in the health professions. Abingdon: Radcliffe Publishing Ltd.; 2013.

Center for Creative Leadership White Paper. Addressing the leadership gap in healthcare: what's needed when it comes to leader talent?. 2011. http://www.ccl.org/leadership/pdf/research/addressingLeadershipGapHealthcare.pdf. Accessed 15 July 2012.

Dannels SA, Yamagata H, McDade SA, Chuang Y, Gleason KA, McLaughlin JA, Richman RC, Morahan PS. Evaluating a leadership program: a comparative, longitudinal study to assess the impact of the Executive Leadership in Academic Medicine (ELAM) Program for women. Acad Med. 2008;83(5):488–95.

McDade SA, Richman RC, Jackson GB, Morahan PS. Effects of participation in the Executive Leadership in Academic Medicine (ELAM) Program on women faculty's perceived leadership capabilities. Acad Med. 2004;79(4):302–9.

Chapter 8
The Business and Finance of Surgical Education

C. Max Schmidt, Laura Torbeck, Heidi Gibbs, and Gary Dunnington

Introduction

Surgical education is the process by which knowledge of the surgical discipline is conferred to an individual surgical trainee. Traditionally, trainees are medical students, residents, and fellows. Faculty are typically characterized as educators or trainers but, importantly, must also retrain and be trainees at various times in their careers.

Surgical education, although critically important to the viability of United States healthcare, runs counter to the business of medicine where the bottom line is efficiency and profit. Commercialization of academic medical centers makes this even more difficult, i.e., the difference between academic medicine and private medical practice is increasingly blurred as both are held to the same procedural volume-based standards and incentives.

Optimization of surgical education is dynamic, not static. It must be constantly evolving to incorporate new technological advances and discoveries and meet the changing demands on future surgeons and the needs of our patients. Thus, more than any other medical specialty, surgical education requires a significant investment of time, effort, money, and resources. The total cost of surgical education is

---

C.M. Schmidt, MD, PhD, MBA, FACS (✉)
Department of Surgery, Indiana University School of Medicine,
980 W Walnut St R3-C522, Indianapolis, IN 46202, USA
e-mail: maxschmi@iupui.edu

L. Torbeck, PhD • H. Gibbs, CPA, MBA • G. Dunnington, MD, FACS
Department of Surgery, Indiana University School of Medicine,
545 Barnhill Drive, Indianapolis, IN 46202, USA

C.M. Pugh, R.S. Sippel (eds.), *Success in Academic Surgery:*
Developing a Career in Surgical Education, Success in Academic Surgery,
DOI 10.1007/978-1-4471-4691-9_8, © Springer-Verlag London 2013

shared by multiple groups including the federal government (Medicare/Medicaid, Department of Defense, Veterans Administration), insurers, industry, hospitals, universities (medical school, surgery department), patients, and trainees/students.

The most important component of surgical education is a conducive learning environment. Such an environment must be consistent across the school of medicine, the department of surgery, and the program's affiliated hospitals. In a conducive environment, even service obligations become educational opportunities. In addition to a conducive environment, key components of surgical education include a dedicated and committed faculty, students willing to learn, and resources to facilitate learning.

Faculty, in addition to having a personal interest in surgical education, should also be incentivized by various mechanisms, monetary and nonmonetary, within the system optimally by the school, department, and hospital. Students' willingness to learn should be fostered in the system by faculty mentoring as well as minimizing the student's conflicting obligations (or a perception of conflicting obligations), e.g., service. Finally, in addition to the hospital's patient care resources, a skills lab to facilitate animate and inanimate/virtual learning is optimal. Faculty incentives, minimizing student's conflicting service obligations, and costs of equipment, animals, and disposables, as well as lost service time of a skills lab will all run counter to the business of academic medicine where academic surgeon compensation is based on patient procedural volume.

Cost of Surgical Education

Surgical education is enormously expensive. In the current era of Medicare/Medicaid funding of GME, resident and fellow salaries are covered. Thus, the costs of surgical education include personnel costs of full- and part-time educators, costs of administrative infrastructure necessary to support this mission, and any costs of the actual educational curriculum. One of the most costly investments in surgical education is the development of ongoing support of a surgical skills laboratory. A surgical skills lab will also include expendable (e.g., gowns, gloves, drugs, anesthesia/surgical disposables, and animals), space, and capital expenditure costs to purchase equipment, equipment updates, and maintenance. The American College of Surgeons has provided very clear guidelines regarding square footage, necessary personnel, administrative infrastructure, and curriculum for the establishment of a surgical skills laboratory. Meeting these requirements allows a skills laboratory to be accredited at either a level I or level II status. The initial outlay can be in the range of one to two million dollars depending on the size of residency and the sophistication of the skills laboratory. These costs include not only costs for building out the facility but operating room like lighting, laparoscopic towers, surgical instruments, and very expensive virtual reality devices.

The total cost of surgical education is shared by multiple groups including the federal government (Medicare/Medicaid, Department of Defense, Veterans Administration), insurers, industry, hospitals, universities (medical school, surgery department), patients, and trainees/students. Similar to the mission of surgical research, it is at best a "break even" budget item.

In the past, the cost of graduate surgical education was born by hospitals which built these costs into patient charges. Over time, however, this was no longer sustainable, as graduate medical education (GME) eventually became the norm (and the standard) rather than the exception. In response, the federal government provided direct (DGME) funding through Medicare to cover resident physician salaries/benefits, faculty compensation, and administrative costs. Ultimately, indirect (IME) funding was also provided by Medicare to cover the increased costs of teaching hospitals including greater inefficiencies, lower payer mix, higher patient acuity (case mix), and state-of-the-art technology. A disproportionate share hospital (DSH) payment adjustment was also provided to cover the variability of indigent patient care.

IME funding was significantly decreased in 1997 with the Balanced Budget Act. In the face of rising GME costs, many teaching hospitals suffered significant losses. Congress ceased further reductions of IME funding, but federal support of GME continues to be a subject of intense debate. Several agencies including the US Department of Health and Human Services Council on Graduate Medical Education (COGME), the Medicare Payment Advisory Commission (Med-PAC), the House Energy and Commerce Subcommittee on Health, the Association of American Medical Colleges, the National Commission on Fiscal Responsibility and Reform (NCFRR), the US Congressional Budget Office (CBO), the Institute of Medicine (IOM), and the Research and Development Corporation (RAND) continue to debate the appropriate extent, allocation, and use of federal and state funding of GME. Several of these agencies have recently proposed cuts in GME. For example, Med-PAC proposed reduction of IME payment from 5.5 to 2.2 %. The NCFRR likewise supported a proposed reduction of IME payment to 2.2 %. Several congressional acts have been introduced to limit IME including the All-Payer Graduate Medical Education Act and the Medical Education Trust Fund Act. Both of these sought to spread some of the burdens of GME to private payers. The Super Committee on Deficit Reduction failed to reach consensus on GME funding and thus, due to sequestration, will result in a cut of GME over the next 10 years by 2 %. President Obama's budget proposals also sought to reduce GME funding. The 2012 budget proposed elimination of $317 million of pediatric GME funding, and the 2013 proposal called for elimination of $88 million of pediatric GME and an IME reduction by $9.7 billion over the next 10 years.

Currently, the bulk of funding for GME is through Medicare. Medicare funds residency programs and teaching hospitals $9.5 billion/year for GME. Of this, $3 billion of DGME is provided to residency programs to cover approximately 100,000 residency positions. The $6.5 billion is provided through IME directly to teaching hospitals. There are many problems with the current system of Medicare funding. These include interinstitutional variability, inter-specialty variability, outdated cost recalibration, physician educator control of direct medical education (DGME) funds is inconsistent, and institutional IME payments unrelated to expenditures for GME or programmatic outcomes. A reanalysis of true cost of GME (including adjustments for local market factors) is needed. DGME optimally should go directly to the physician organization providing resident education. Budget and expenditures for GME should be tracked and reported, and GME program performance standards should be established. Failure to achieve performance standards should result in loss of funds.

Medicaid funds teaching hospitals $3.78 billion/year for GME. These payments are structured in large part similar to Medicare GME funds. The difference is that Medicaid funds are state government derived. There is no obligation on the part of states to provide funding of GME through Medicaid. As state government budgets get tighter, many states are opting to default on payment for Medicaid. This will put increased pressure on alternative sources of GME funding.

The trainees/students fund their own education through tuition payments and billing for services provided. Medical student payments of tuition to the school of medicine help defray the personnel costs of medical school faculty and in some cases surgical faculty. Although graduate medical education is typically funded by the federal government, fellows are typically only partially covered. Fellows with a faculty appointment may provide billable services which may help defray the costs of surgical education.

If federal government funding of GME falters, revenues from surgical education will need to come from hospitals. Teaching hospitals, however, are already financially weak and education missions are stressed. The cause of this is multifactorial including rapidly changing medical technology, decreased reimbursement for service, increased uncompensated care, increased wage costs, and reductions in federal GME payments. If hospitals pay for GME in this environment, the cost will inevitably be passed on to insurers and ultimately patients.

Department Budget

The department budget includes all expenses and revenues of the department. The department supports the missions of service, teaching, and research. Each of these missions has associated expenses and revenues.

Most expenses and revenues originate from a particular division and thus can be easily assigned to a particular division within the department of surgery. As such, these can be handled according to the division. In general, a division's revenues should largely cover its expenses, such that each unit is responsible for its own budget. The clinical mission, in particular, is ideally suited for divisions handling the resulting revenues and expenses. Money flows into the divisions from the practice plan and hospital according to the division's clinical productivity. This is similar for the mission of research. Clinical trial revenue and research grant support flow into the divisions from which the trial or grant originated. Any recovery of indirect costs of grants should also return to the division from which the grant originated. Similarly, for any committee or other service to the school which is compensated, the individual and/or division performing the service should receive the revenues.

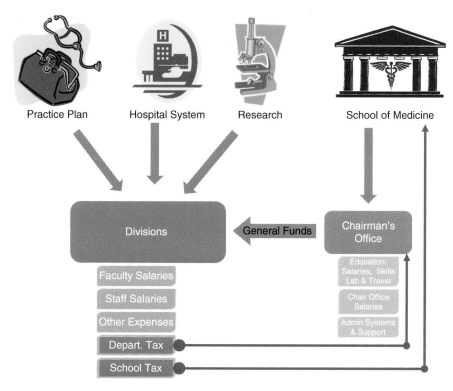

Fig. 8.1 Department of surgery funds flow: revenues from clinical service (practice plan, hospital system) and research flow into the department. Clinical practice and research revenues will largely be credited to the particular division within the department from which they are generated to cover expenses of these activities. Some divisional expenses, however, are not directly related to the missions of clinical service and research. The school's (or dean's) tax and department tax are examples of such expenses which flow out of the divisions to the school of medicine and the department, respectively. The school's tax supports the activities of the dean's office, whereas the department tax helps support the chairman's office and any activities which are thought to be in the collective interest of the department. Surgical education is one of these activities. Surgical education is also subsidized through government and private funds transferred from the school of medicine to the department

Some divisional expenses are not directly related to the missions of service and research. The dean's tax and department tax are examples of such expenses which flow out of the divisions to the school of medicine and the department respectively (Fig. 8.1). The dean's tax supports the activities of the dean's office, whereas the department tax helps support the chairman's office and any activities which are thought to be in the collective interest of the department. One example of this would be salaries for surgical residents in research fellowship.

In contrast to the missions of service and research, the mission of education does not lend itself as well to division support. This is in part because different divisions may contribute unequally to the educational mission. Regardless, the educational mission must be strongly supported by the department. Education expenses and revenues, therefore, should be shared by all of the divisions since it is a core component of the overall department mission. The main sources of revenue for surgical education as noted previously come to the department through the school of medicine (subsidized from federal/state government and medical school tuition). The department of surgery distributes federal/state government and tuition revenues to support the educational costs (administrative, faculty, and nonfaculty support) and salaries of residents/fellows. The school of medicine funds distributed to the department are shown in Fig. 8.2a. The school of medicine distributes these funds equitably according to the relative contribution of the division in resident/fellow education and medical student education as shown in Fig. 8.2b. Department of surgery financial spreadsheets (balance sheet and income statement) are also included to facilitate understanding of the scope of the educational costs relative to overall department budget (Table 8.1a, b).

Funding the Educational Mission and Surgical Educators

Funding the educational mission and your surgical educators should be transparent, rational, and mutually acceptable. Creative approaches and solutions to financing surgical education are needed, so we can maintain the viability of the system to produce a high-quality surgeon work force trained to address the public needs.

Because education often runs counter to the business of academic medicine, educators need to be incentivized and have any obvious barriers removed. This ideally occurs throughout the entire healthcare system including the school of medicine, surgery department, and any affiliated hospitals. While there are a number of programs that have published their experience, most rely on withholding of a certain percentage of clinical receipts for redistribution to faculty based on the accumulated credits in areas such as teaching or research. Such a program allows busy clinical faculty to still contribute to the educational mission by providing funds that can support those with significant commitment in educational leadership or skills laboratory activities. Another option is to create a faculty withhold of one to two dollars per RVU produced to fund the educational mission. While these methods clearly place an additional burden on clinical practice to subsidize education, it is likely that this will need to be a component of the overall educational budget.

In addition to incentives for educators, creative approaches and solutions to financing surgical education are needed. What follows are some ideas to fund the educational mission and surgical educators:

1. Faculty fellows may bill for services. Revenues from billings for their services should directly benefit the division the fellow is being trained in.
2. Educational research grants (e.g., NIH, AHRQ, Association for Surgical Education) may help support the educational mission by defraying the costs of

a

Grouping	Allocation Type	FY2013 Sum of Allocation ($)	Allocation based on:
Directed Allocation	Chair Supplement	75,000.00	Standard Chair Support
	Department Fixed Admin	100,000.00	Standard Administration Support
	Faculty Rent Credit	200,000.00	Based on $ per number of faculty
Directed Allocation subtotal		375,000.00	
Education	Residents & Fellows	845,000.00	Based on $ per number of Residents & Fellows
	Student Fees Med Stud Clerkships	1,250,000.00	Based on # of clerkship weeks
	Student Fees Med Stud Clerkships Over Sight	150,000.00	Based on clerkship at all sites (Clerkship Director & Coordinator)
	Med Student Electives	350,000.00	Based on Elective EVU's (Course length in days x #Students enrolled)
	Student Fee Med Students 1 & 2	25,000.00	Based on Direct contact hours (specific conference, lecture or workshop)
Service To School	Education Committee Service	15,000.00	Specific Committee participation
Education Subtotal		2,635,000.00	
Indirect Recovery (from research grants)		1,015,000.00	Based on 3 yr rolling average of indirects, 2 yrs in arrears, allocated to division of PI
State Directed Allocation Across the Board Reduction		(161,000.00)	Budget cut, based on X% of Direct Allocation + Education + Indirects
Space Rent		(1,035,000.00)	Based on square footage (point in time snapshot)
University Information Technology Bundled Charges		(10,000.00)	University Information Tech Bundled Charges
		2,819,000.00	

b

	Total School Funds	Administration, Chairman and Medical Education	Cardiac Surgery	General Surgery	Pediatric Surgery	Plastic Surgery	Transplant Surgery	Vascular Surgery
Administrative Allocation								
Chair Admin Stipend	75,000	75,000						
Standard Dept. Admin Allocation	100,000	100,000						
Faculty Rent Credit	200,000	10,000	25,000	80,000	20,000	25,000	20,000	20,000
	375,000	185,000	25,000	80,000	20,000	25,000	20,000	20,000
Education Allocation	2,635,000	725,000	250,000	900,000	210,000	200,000	175,000	175,000
	2,635,000	725,000	250,000	900,000	210,000	200,000	175,000	175,000
Indirect Allocation (Faculty Effort by Investigator 3 year rolling average)	1,015,000	300,000	25,000	500,000	25,000	25,000	15,000	125,000
	1,015,000	300,000	25,000	500,000	25,000	25,000	15,000	125,000
UITS Bundled (University Information Technology Services)	(10,000)	(10,000)						
State Directed Reduction –4%	(161,000)	(48,400)	(12,000)	(59,200)	(10,200)	(10,000)	(8,400)	(12,800)
	(171,000)	(58,400)	(12,000)	(59,200)	(10,200)	(10,000)	(8,400)	(12,800)
Faculty Endow Match (per Gift Agreements)		165,000	(15,000)	(50,000)	(25,000)	(25,000)	(25,000)	(25,000)
Stipends		(310,000)	15,000	175,000	50,000	50,000	10,000	10,000
Total Allocation Before Space Costs FY 2013	$ 3,854,000	$ 1,006,600	$ 288,000	$ 1,545,800	$ 269,800	$ 265,000	$ 186,600	$ 292,200
Space Allocation	(1,035,000)	(225,000)	(90,000)	(300,000)	(75,000)	(125,000)	(125,000)	(95,000)
Net Total General Funds Allocation	$ 2,819,000	$ 781,600	$ 198,000	$ 1,245,800	$ 194,800	$ 140,000	$ 61,600	$ 197,200

Fig. 8.2 The school of medicine funds (**a**) distributed to the department are shown. The school of medicine distributes these funds equitably according to the relative contribution of the division in resident/fellow education and medical student education (**b**)

Table 8.1 (a) Balance Sheet

Surgeons Incorporated
Balance Sheet
12/31/XX

	Current Year 12/31/XX Actual	Prior Year 12/31/XX Actual
Assets		
Current Assets		
Cash	$3,693,000	$2,600,000
Total Current Assets	3,693,000	2,600,000
Property & Equipment		
Fixed Assets	175,000	125,000
Accum. Dep.	(125,000)	(115,000)
Other Assets		
Intangibles	15,000	15,000
Accum. Amortization	(5,000)	(5,000)
Net Other Assets	10,000	10,000
Total Assets	$3,753,000	$2,620,000
Liabilities		
Short Term Liabiliaties	350,000	400,000
Other Liabilities	1,750,000	1,450,000
Total Liabilities	2,100,000	1,850,000
Equity		
Common Stock	100	100
Retained Earnings	159,900	119,900
Dividend Payment	(450,000)	(350,000)
Current Year Earnings	1,943,000	1,000,000
Total Equity	1,653,000	770,000
Total Liabilities and Equity	$3,753,000	$2,620,000

Table 8.1 (b) Income Statement

Surgeons Incorporated
Income Statement
For the Twelve Months Ending December 31, 20XX

	Month Ending 12/31/XX Total	Year-to-date 12/31/XX Total
Revenue		
Professional Fees	4,200,000	54,000,000
Refunds	(116,000)	(1,500,000)
Call Coverage	250,000	3,000,000
Medical Directorship	150,000	1,800,000
Contract Income	12,000	115,000
Other Income	32,000	450,000
Total Revenue	$ 4,528,000	$ 57,865,000
Expenses		
Physician & Academic Salary	2,700,000	31,500,000
Physician & Academic Fringe Bbenefits	810,000	9,450,000
Professional & Admistrative Salary	260,000	2,850,000
Professional & Adminsitrative Fringe Benefits	72,800	798,000
Pension Contribution	50,000	650,000
Billing Fees	163,360	2,100,000
Travel & Meals	70,000	1,120,000
Dues, Subscriptons, Books, License	25,000	225,000
Research Supplies	75,000	895,000
School, System, & Department Taxes	425,000	5,500,000
Bank Charges	3,250	39,000
Software, Technology & Computer Expense	20,000	200,000
Copies/Printing	2,500	30,000
Freight/Hauling/ Postage	2,500	30,000
Medical & Surgical Supplies	1,000	15,000
Miscellaneous Expense	10,000	200,000
Office Supplies	2,500	30,000
Recruiting	5,000	75,000
Repairs & Maintenance	2,500	30,000
Resident & Student Expenses	8,000	100,000
Storage	2,000	25,000
Telephone	2,000	25,000
Visual Media & Advertising	2,000	50,000
Total Expenses	$ 4,714,410	$ 55,937,000
Operating Income	$ (186,410)	$ 1,928,000
Other Income (Expense)		
Interest Income	1,000	15,000
Total Other Income (Expense)	$ 1,000	$ 15,000
Net Income	$ (185,410)	$ 1,943,000

salaries of surgery faculty, non-surgeon faculty, and educators. Grants may also help fund capital costs of surgical skills laboratories.

3. Endowments, if available at the department or university level, may be able to help fund surgical education in part through endowment funds.
4. Establish a departmental reserve fund may be useful in planning for deficits in GME funding, particularly in the absence of an endowment.
5. Industry may be able to help fund education, particularly surgical skills labs since the sustenance of these labs helps preserve the safety of our patients. Conflict of interest policies, however, has constrained some of these relationships considerably making it ever more difficult to receive unrestricted funds in the absence of significant acknowledgement of the source of industry funds.
6. A reduction of time of residency, e.g., general surgery. A quicker transition to subspecialty training where faculty fellows may bill for services may be necessary to help afford GME in the absence of federal funding.
7. Reductions in low utilization services and mid-level providers may be necessary to afford to fund GME.

Surgical skills labs are becoming increasingly utilized to optimize surgical education and promote safe surgery. This is a unique cost of surgical education. The following suggestions are provided to assist departments in both the initial implementation of a skills laboratory and in maintaining ongoing budgets:

1. Create a multidisciplinary venture with partnerships with other surgical specialty departments as well as departments such as emergency medicine and OBGYN. Ongoing operating costs can be shared across multiple departments with calculation of each department's costs by percentage of total use. By necessity, this will require the creation of a management board that includes leadership from all participating departments.
2. Create a partnership with the hospital or healthcare plan with the venture identified as a clear patient safety initiative. There is now ample evidence to show that surgical trainees spending time in a surgical skills laboratory have enhanced performance in the operating room with less operative time, decreased errors, and improved patient outcome. Hospital investment in a skills laboratory is further warranted as a critical expenditure for recruitment of high-quality candidates to the training program. If ongoing basic expenditures can be covered by participating departments, hospitals can play a significant role in the purchase of expensive virtual reality devices, particularly when a business plan can be presented for widespread users and a direct benefit to trainee performance in patient settings.
3. The surgical skills laboratory provides an excellent opportunity for major philanthropy for possible naming rights. The partnership with school of medicine development staff can provide opportunities to share the vision of how surgical skills laboratory is shaping the future training of surgeons to potential donors, including retired surgeons and industry.

Formal Education in Business (MBA) and Education (Master's, PhD)

Leaders of surgical education should have an excellent working knowledge of business as well as education. Knowledge of both business and education can be obtained through a combination of experience, formal education, and/or a highly experienced/educated staff who can work closely with the surgeon leader. It is important for a leader of surgical education to understand reimbursement, charity care, cost of doing business, benchmarking, accounting standards, and ethics. It is also important to know how to generate new business and/or increase market share to support growth and increased capacity of the educational programming. Formal courses that deal with these important aspects include accounting, finance, management, and marketing/development. The importance of an MBA versus a Master's or PhD in surgical education depends more on the physician's role and long-term goals and objectives. An MBA will provide knowledge on how a business runs and key tools for marketing, benchmarking, cost analysis, accounting, and leadership skills. A Master's or PhD in surgical education will put more emphasis on educating students and residents and leadership skills. Each of these chosen advanced degrees will provide different tools to the learner. They should not be considered mutually exclusive degrees as both could be highly beneficial to obtain. Formal degrees in business and education could significantly enhance a surgeon leader's ability to effectively manage a surgical education program. Nonetheless, while desirable, formal degrees in business and education are definitely not a necessity for the success of surgical education leaders. A dedicated and committed leader supported by individuals with formal knowledge of business, education, and the practice of surgery can also be a formula for success of a surgical education program.

Summary

Surgical education must continue to be promoted to the highest level for the public good. The resources required for surgical education are immense. To meet this need is challenging in an environment where surgical education runs counter to the business of academic medicine. This is further challenged by the decline in government support of graduate medical education. The business and finance of surgical education has become quite complex. Programs will need to reinvent themselves to thrive. Surgical education should have strong advocacy, experienced and educated leaders, incentivized faculty, a skilled staff with formal education in business and education, and multiple and creative approaches to financing surgical education.

Further Reading

Mallon WT, Jones RF, Mallon WT, Jones RF. How do medical schools use measurement systems to track faculty activity and productivity in teaching? Acad Med. 2002;77:115–23.

Metzler I, Ganjawalla K, Kaups KL, Meara JG. The critical state of graduate medical education funding. Bull Am Coll Surg. 2012;97(11):9–18.

Rich EC, Liebow M, Srinivasan M, Parish D, Wolliscroft JO, Fein O, Blaser R. Medicare financing of graduate medical education. J Gen Intern Med. 2002;17(4):283–92.

Sites S, Vansaghi L, Pingleton S, Cox G, Paolo A. Aligning compensation with education: design and implementation of the educational value unit (EVU) system in an academic internal medicine department. Acad Med. 2005;80(12):1100–6.

Williams R, Dunnington G, Folse R. The impact of a program for systematically recognizing and rewarding academic performance. Acad Med. 2003;78(2):156–66.

Chapter 9
Mentors and Mentoring

Nicholas R. Teman and Rebecca M. Minter

Introduction

The origin of the term mentor comes from Homer's *The Odyssey*, in which the character Mentor was entrusted to care for Telemachus, the son of Odysseus. When Odysseus left Greece to fight in the Trojan War, he placed Mentor in charge of raising his son. Mentor cultivated a relationship with Telemachus through guidance and education and came to treat him much like a son. It is this type of relationship and support that has come to be the idealized form of modern mentorship. As one publication noted, "mentoring is about helping people to make their own choices by suggesting options to them. It is not about telling them what to do or how to do it. Mentoring is a developing relationship encompassing a wide range of issues, not just those concerned with problem-solving – career, personal, or family issues may arise. It is imperative, therefore, that a mentor is prepared to think about the broader aspects of people development and the factors that influence them in their daily work and their choice of careers."

Historically, surgery has been a field which is defined by strong mentorship. The Halstedian apprenticeship model of surgical education is essentially that of a mentor-mentee relationship. Trainees would spend years learning surgical techniques, patient care, and life lessons from their elders. Often, these relationships would persist as lifelong learning throughout their careers. Mentorship remains a critical element of surgical training in the current era; however, the classic apprenticeship model has been replaced with a team approach to mentorship. In today's environment of increasing service and time requirements coupled with a lack of resources, it can be difficult to succeed without guidance from a mentor. Several previous authors have noted the difficulty of finding an appropriate mentor in surgery. This

N.R. Teman, MD • R.M. Minter, MD (✉)
Department of Surgery, University of Michigan Health System,
Ann Arbor, MI, USA
e-mail: nteman@med.umich.edu; rminter@umich.edu

C.M. Pugh, R.S. Sippel (eds.), *Success in Academic Surgery:*
Developing a Career in Surgical Education, Success in Academic Surgery,
DOI 10.1007/978-1-4471-4691-9_9, © Springer-Verlag London 2013

can be even more pronounced in the field of surgical education, which has not been as clearly recognized historically as an academic or research focus as compared to basic science or health services research. Though there have been significant gains in recognition of education as a viable career path in academic surgery, the path to success remains somewhat less transparent than for some other areas of scholarship focus. As such, surgeons interested in education often find it difficult to garner sufficient time and resources to pursue their goals. Thus, it is critical to identify a mentor who has been successful in the field of surgical education who can guide the mentee and assist them in ensuring that their work in education is viewed as a valuable academic endeavor and not simply a side activity or hobby.

As in every other aspect of professional development, success in surgical education depends on appropriate guidance from those who have previously blazed the trail. Choosing an appropriate mentor and getting the most out of the mentor-mentee relationship is critical to the development of a career in surgical education. The goal of this chapter is to provide instruction on finding a mentor, getting the most out of a mentor, and subsequently using one's learned skills and experiences to mentor others in the future.

Finding a Mentor

Several important qualities of a good mentor are listed in Table 9.1. Not surprisingly, these are the same qualities that most of us would seek out in a friend, partner, or confidant. Each of these is a valuable trait, but perhaps the most desirable quality is one's motivation and willingness to be a mentor. When trying to identify a mentor, an obvious place to start is to try to identify an individual who has a career that you would aspire to emulate – in this case, a successful surgical educator. This individual must also be someone whom you are comfortable with and who you feel you could forge a relationship with over the course of years. Forcing a connection when the desire is not present is disingenuous and counterproductive. Additionally, it is critical to choose a mentor who is available. The most famous individual is often not the best mentor due to competing demands and lack of sufficient time to really mentor colleagues or trainees. A focus on identifying a mentor who has the time to commit to your development is far more important than their degree of fame.

Table 9.1 Qualities of a good mentor

Accessible	Experienced	Knowledgeable
Approachable	Generous	Motivated
Caring	Honest	Objective
Committed	Humble	Professional
Compassionate	Interested	Respectful
Dedicated	Insightful	Responsible
Empowering	Inspiring	Supportive

There are several considerations unique to finding a mentor in surgical education. The number of people qualified and motivated to be mentors in this field is smaller than other domains of academic surgical practice. While most departments have expert clinicians, for example, not all have experienced surgical educators. Junior faculty and residents interested in education as a scholarship focus are lucky if they have one possible mentor at their institution, let alone several. For this reason, it is often necessary to look outside one's own institution to find a mentor. With current technologies for phone and Internet video conferencing, collaborating across town or across countries has become significantly easier. Motivation and desire are far more important qualities in a mentor than geographical proximity.

Reaching out to contacts on a national level can be an important component of developing a relationship with a mentor. Major national surgical meetings, including the American College of Surgeons Annual Clinical Congress and the Academic Surgical Congress, now have entire sessions dedicated to surgical education. The Association for Surgical Education, Association of Residency Coordinators in Surgery, and Association of Program Directors in Surgery jointly sponsor Surgical Education Week every year. This meeting consists of 6 days of programming specifically intended for those interested in surgical education. The importance of networking and developing relationships at these meetings cannot be understated. One would be hard-pressed to find a larger collection of leaders and innovators in surgical education in a single venue.

Another source for a mentor in surgical education is the Surgical Education Research Fellowship (SERF), sponsored by the Association for Surgical Education (www.surgicaleducation.com/serf-program). This yearlong program consists of two off-site seminars combined with independent learning and the completion of a surgical education project at the Fellow's home institution. A critical component of the Fellowship is the assignment of an advisor who guides the Fellow as they complete their project. This advisor is a nationally recognized leader in surgical education and/or education research. They provide mentorship to the Fellow through frequent communication regarding the project, with the goal of establishing a long-term mutually beneficial relationship. For those interested in surgical education without a mentor available at their institution, this is an excellent option for identifying a mentor.

Another unique aspect of mentoring in surgical education is related to the wide variety of skills needed to be successful. As the breadth of this book demonstrates, surgical education requires a unique and diverse skill set, very little of which is taught during medical school or surgical residency. These skills may include conducting qualitative research, performing statistical analyses specific to education research, understanding education theory, and other specific aspects of education research, such as simulation or psychomotor training. One could envision a "team" of mentors, with expertise in each of these facets of surgical education, and the mentee synthesizing the guidance and experience of these mentors. An example of such a team is shown in Fig. 9.1.

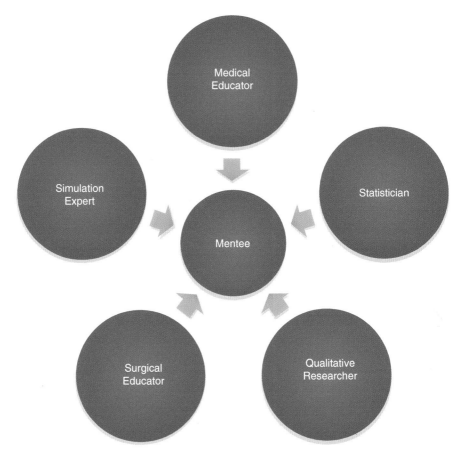

Fig. 9.1 An example of "mentorship by committee," in which the mentee is guided by several individuals, each with a different skill set and area of expertise

Getting the Most Out of Your Mentor

The most important determinant of a successful mentoring relationship is the selection of an appropriate mentor, as described in the previous section. Now that a mentor has been chosen, how can the mentee get the most out of this relationship? The key to maximizing the mentorship experience is to take advantage of the numerous roles that the mentor can fill. A good mentor is simultaneously a teacher, coach, critic, parent, friend, cheerleader, and role model.

Teaching and coaching are perhaps the most important roles of an ideal mentor. Mentors are responsible for imparting the knowledge that they have accrued from their previous experiences. While nothing can replace firsthand experience, mentees should use these interactions as an opportunity to learn from the mentor's successes and failures. Mentors can also help with strategizing to meet the objectives of the mentee. Early in the mentor-mentee relationship, there should be frank discussions regarding the clinical, professional, and academic goals of the mentee. Honesty and insight are critical to avoid wasted time and efforts. The strategy for optimizing the success of a given mentee will be different if he/she wishes to dedicate the majority of their academic time to surgical education versus establishing a busy clinical practice with only a small focus on education. The mentorship approach must be tailored to the needs of the mentee and the skills of their mentor; a "one size fits all" method is doomed to fail.

To that end, it is critical that the mentee be completely honest with their mentor regarding their goals and aspirations, even if quite different from the path their mentor has followed. It is dangerous and disingenuous to try and please your mentor by giving the impression that you are interested in a topic or career path for which you are not passionate, and it is important that the mentee is true to himself/herself in working with a mentor to define their own personal vision and goals. Simply becoming a carbon copy of a mentor is not the goal and will limit a mentee's ability to be maximally effective in his/her own life's work.

As noted, one will likely have many mentors who provide guidance in different aspects of one's personal and professional life. It is important to consider what assistance a mentee would like from a given mentor so that they may work towards that goal together. Mismatched expectations create conflict within the relationship and limit ultimate success. Once the mentee and mentor's goals and expectations are aligned, creating an action plan with a timeline for specific milestones will help to keep both the mentee and mentor accountable in the relationship.

Occasionally, one will select a mentor that is not a good fit. This can occur for a variety of reasons – a mentor who is too busy to provide guidance and assistance to their mentee, a poor personality fit, or a shift in the interests and direction of the mentee. Should this occur, the best path forward is honest acknowledgement that the mentor-mentee relationship is not working, and if the gap cannot be bridged, then identification of a new mentor is appropriate.

Mentoring Others

The mentor-mentee relationship should be a balance of challenge and support. Communication and trust should be such that the mentor can provide honest constructive criticism. However, this can be a difficult balance to strike. Too much challenging can stifle development of the mentee, but too much support without appropriate challenging precludes critical thinking and introspection which is necessary for development. The mentor and mentee each have obligations to the process if it is to be successful. Responsibilities of a mentor include a strong commitment; giving the mentee access to their experience, contacts, and wealth of knowledge; encouraging and supporting the mentee's professional endeavors; providing feedback which is specific and constructive; challenging and stimulating the mentee to achieve additional success; and acknowledging the mentee's contributions and successes. The mentee, on the other hand, must approach the mentor with an open mind, be willing to listen to criticism as well as praise, emulate the positive characteristics of the mentor, and acknowledge the contributions and support of the mentor. If a successful mentor-mentee relationship is established and optimized, both mentee and mentor will derive great benefit.

In mentoring others, it is critical that one is generous with their time and honest with oneself in only accepting a mentee if they can make the time available to provide the guidance needed. The mentee must be accountable and follow through on planned deliverables just as the mentor must be a finisher as well. There is nothing more frustrating to a mentee than waiting for a mentor to provide feedback on a manuscript or other work product that they have invested significant time and effort into completing. A mentor must "lead from the front" and exemplify the behavior that they would like to see in their mentees in terms of work ethic and productivity, while also holding their mentees accountable and pushing them towards independence.

In mentoring others within the field of surgical education, it is critical that the mentor exposes the mentee to the broad array of resources available and necessary for success in this field, not just their own expertise. Additionally, given the relative paucity of surgical educators at many institutions as compared to experts in other fields of academic surgery, distance mentoring is not uncommon. As a mentor or leader in the field of surgical education, one should be open to mentoring junior faculty and residents from other institutions. These relationships will serve to build a network of successful surgical educators across multiple sites, which will greatly benefit the field of surgical education as a whole.

In summary, establishing an optimal mentor-mentee relationship is a mutual effort, and both parties will derive significant benefit if these relationships are ideally constructed. It is critically important that both the mentor and mentee are completely clear on their expectations and goals for the relationship and that these are clearly communicated. If the relationship is established with this framework as the foundation, then the potential for success and great personal reward for both mentor and mentee is limitless.

Further Reading

Memon B, Memon MA. Mentoring and surgical training: a time for reflection! Adv Health Sci Educ Theory Pract. 2010;15:749–54.

Patel VM, Warren O, Ahmed K, et al. How can we build mentorship in surgeons of the future? ANZ J Surg. 2011;81:418–24.

Ramani S, Gruppen L, Kachur EK. Twelve tips for developing effective mentors. Med Teach. 2006;28:404–8.

Sosa JA. Choosing, and being, a good mentor. In: Chen H, Kao LS, editors. Success in academic surgery. London: Springer; 2012. p. 169–80.

Souba WW. Mentoring young academic surgeons, our most precious asset. J Surg Res. 1999;82:113–20.

Chapter 10
Training Opportunities in Medical and Surgical Education

Brenessa Lindeman and Stephen C. Yang

As a surgeon, the requirement for academic clinical practice is completion of an accredited residency program with or without a fellowship, followed by appropriate board certification. It was classically assumed that those who complete this rigorous training process in an academic setting naturally developed the teaching skills necessary to teach the next generation of academic surgeons. To date, no specific training paradigm has been defined for individuals desiring to become surgical educators. Historically, volunteer academic faculty have shouldered the responsibility of teaching medical students and residents with little to no additional insights beyond what they were exposed to during their own curriculum. Unfortunately, their teaching commitments were sometimes viewed as a distraction from the tasks of grant application and publication of research efforts. With the added pressures of research and clinical productivity, the ability and the time dedicated to teaching have been placed low on the prioritization of academic tasks. The "student" generational gap has changed since most of us have trained, as educational technology and techniques have evolved to capture the attention of our trainees.

A growing body of knowledge has broadened the definition of scholarship, and an increasing number of academic health centers recognize education scholarship in their tenure and promotion process, some with creation of a "clinician-educator" track. The modern conception of scholarship has centered on common criteria for its identification: clear goals, adequate preparation, appropriate methods, significant results, effective presentation, and reflective critique [1]. This chapter will focus on how to achieve the second of the Glassick criteria – adequate preparation. It begins with seeking out opportunities for dedicated training in the field one hopes to pursue and will require the investment of time to bring to fruition. In surgical education, optimal training opportunities should be designed to provide at least the basic skills

B. Lindeman, MD • S.C. Yang, MD (✉)
Department of Surgery, The Johns Hopkins Medical Institutions,
Baltimore, MD, USA
e-mail: b.lindeman@jhmi.edu; syang@jhmi.edu

C.M. Pugh, R.S. Sippel (eds.), *Success in Academic Surgery:*   81
Developing a Career in Surgical Education, Success in Academic Surgery,
DOI 10.1007/978-1-4471-4691-9_10, © Springer-Verlag London 2013

necessary to become an effective teacher, leader, and administrator in surgical education programs. For some individuals, structured opportunities within their residency training may provide this requisite educational experience with medical students and residents, but the majority of surgeons will need to complete additional focused training to become qualified surgical educators.

Generally, all medical schools have an office in faculty development that offers basic courses in medical education such as curriculum development, assessment, and feedback. Centers with specific academic educator tracks also provide support either through formal courses or through internal Web links. This role of education has even filtered to the medical student level, wherein the basic concept of curriculum development has been introduced as a longitudinal track of interested medical students at certain institutions.

A wide variety of training opportunities for those interested in medical education currently exist. These exist in various forms in length, formality, and availability. Some are given catchy program titles such as "Teach the Teacher," "Educate the Educator," or "Train the Trainer." Those targeted specifically to the surgical field include the "Surgical Education Research Fellowship" sponsored by the Association for Surgical Education and the "Surgeons as Educators" course from the American College of Surgeons. Multiple other educator development courses such as those sponsored by the Harvard Macy Institute or the Association for American Medical Colleges, as well as national and international medical education fellowships, exist for the entire population of medical educators. A partial list is outlined in Table 10.1. Specialty-specific programs and courses have been introduced such as "Educate the Educator" for the field of cardiothoracic surgery. Additionally, the new field of simulation education and training has emerged, and a number of simulation medicine fellowships have been created at academic health centers across the country in response.

Surgery-Specific Opportunities

Surgeons as Educators Course

Almost 20 years ago, the American College of Surgeons recognized the need to support surgeons in leadership roles at residency training programs with instruction in basic educational knowledge and skills. They responded with the creation of the Surgeons as Educators course, a 6-day on-site experience designed to foster the unique skill set of teachers and administrators of surgical education programs (http://www.facs.org/education/sre/saeintro.html).

The target audience for the course includes academic hospital faculty interested in "acquiring or honing skills in curriculum development, teaching, performance and program evaluation, and program administration and/or who have direct teaching responsibilities for medical students and residents." The course is limited to a maximum of 32 participants.

Table 10.1 Summary of training opportunities in surgical education

Curriculum	Specific program examples	Sponsoring organization
Immersion courses	Surgeons as Educators	ACS
	The Program for Educators in Health Professions, The Leading Innovations in Health Care and Education Program, and A Systems Approach to Assessment in Health Professions Education	Harvard Macy Institute
	Educate the Educators	JCTSE
	Essential Skills in Medical Education	AMEE
Faculty development courses at national meetings	Surgical Education	ACS Fall Clinical Congress
	Surgery Clerkship Director Course	ASE Annual Meeting
	Faculty Development Workshop	APDS Annual Meeting
Sponsored fellowship	Surgical Education Research Fellowship	ASE
	International Fellowship in Medical Education	FAIMER
	Medical Education Fellowship	IAMSE
	Academy for Innovation in Medical Education	AIME/uOSSC
Simulation opportunities	SimPORTAL Simulation Fellowship	University of Minnesota
	Simulation Instructorship Program	Northwestern University
	Schwartz-Reisman Fellowship in Simulation Medicine	Mayo Clinic

Abbreviations: *ACS* American College of Surgeons, *AIME* Academy for Innovation in Medical Education, *AMEE* Association for Medical Education in Europe, *APDS* Association of Program Directors in Surgery, *ASE* Association for Surgical Education, *FAIMER* Foundation for Advancement of International Medical Education and Research, *JCTSE* Joint Council on Thoracic Surgery Education, *IAMSE* International Association of Medical Science Educators, *uOSSC* University of Ottawa Skills and Simulation Center

Curriculum for the course focuses on four broad topics within education: teaching skills, curriculum development, educational administration and leadership, and performance and program evaluation. Instruction in teaching skills is centered on adult learning theory and addresses specific techniques to foster an effective learning environment for medical student, resident, and other health professional learners. Discussions center on application of specific teaching methods and technologies to maximize learning, as well as the administration of an educational program including motivating faculty, implementing change, and managing conflict. Participants are exposed to a number of practical techniques in engaging the learner, as opposed to the classic lecture style. Course participants also engage in the generative work of mapping out an instructional unit such as a clerkship or residency rotation using a provided framework and developing a valid system to assess teacher and learner performance.

Tuition for the course covers all materials, lodging, meals and refreshments, and a welcome reception. The course faculty are national leaders in surgical education; they volunteer for this unselfishly and have consistently produced a flawless program since its existence. It is conducted annually, usually in early to mid-September, and the application process is quite competitive, as there is usually a backlog of faculty who wish to attend. Additional information is available via the American College of Surgeons (ACS) website and through commonly used search engines. Oftentimes, the ACS does put on a 1-day abbreviated course at the Fall Clinical Congress.

This course is considered the preeminent entry point of any surgeon from any specialty to enter the realm of surgical education. Some of the many advantages for attending this program include: (1) exposure to leaders in surgical education who are dedicated in nurturing and mentoring those attendees who wish to pursue education as a career, (2) a concentrated and focused time away from the home clinical practice to immerse oneself into this area, (3) the ability to develop the skills of team building and collegiality outside one's normal environment amongst peers who share the same passion in education, (4) the networking environment in initiating career-long relationships amongst colleagues in the same administrative capacity such as clerkship or program training directors, and (5) the long-term follow-up the course directors provide in tracking your educational program development.

Surgical Education Research Fellowship (SERF)

Led by the Foundation of the Association for Surgical Education, this popular program selects up to 16 individuals with interest in surgical education for a 1-year mentored research experience (http://www.surgicaleducation.com/serf-program). Unique to SERF, participants remain at their homesite for the duration of their work. The program begins with an introductory workshop at the Association for Surgical Education Annual Meeting to provide basic foundational knowledge and skills needed to conduct, apply, and report educational research. At this meeting, participants also brainstorm and refine potential project ideas. Following this session, fellows are carefully matched with an advisor, a well-reputed and knowledgeable researcher, to serve as a mentor and consultant for their project. A second seminar is held at the American College of Surgeons Clinical Congress in the fall, where fellows are expected to give a progress report on their projects.

The goals of SERF fellows completing this program are to be able to access and review the surgical education research literature, design an educational research project using appropriate methodologies, translate the research into academic presentations and/or publications, and establish a network of surgical education research colleagues. To receive a course completion certificate, fellows are expected to collaborate with their advisor on the design and development of the project and submit an abstract or paper either coauthored or approved by their advisor to a peer-reviewed forum or journal. Fellows are typically expected to complete these requirements in 1 year; however, the length of time granted may vary based on the type of project conducted. For example, studies involving larger sample sizes, instrument development, or more sophisticated experimental studies may have up to 3 years to complete the fellowship.

Applicants to the program must be members of the Association for Surgical Education, but residents are encouraged to apply. At the time of press, tuition is $1700.00, plus the cost of the textbook. Other costs include expenses to travel to the two seminars and SERF forum.

International Scholarships for Surgical Education

For young faculty members from institutions outside the United States or Canada, the American College of Surgeons awards two scholarships focused on training in surgical education. These awards from the Divisions of Education and International Relations provide the opportunity to participate in a variety of programs focused on faculty development and acquisition of knowledge and skills with a goal to enhance surgical education and training in their home country (http://www.facs.org/memberservices/issurged.html).

Program participants will attend the American College of Surgeons Clinical Congress and the Surgical Education: Principles and Practice course, as well as plenary sessions addressing topics pertinent to surgical education and training. Following the Clinical Congress, the scholars will visit appropriate Level I ACS-Accredited Education Institutes for exposure to areas aligned with the individual's particular education-based interest. At the completion of their travel, scholars are required to submit a letter to the International Relations Committee delineating the outcomes achieved as a result of the scholarship.

Application requirements for the scholarship include graduation from a school of medicine, age between 30 and 45 years, and practicing surgery for a minimum of 5 years after completion of all formal training. A completed typewritten application in English, plus three letters of recommendation including one from the department chair in support of the scholar's desired educational objectives are required. If unsuccessful, individuals may submit up to two reapplications with new supporting documentation.

Nonspecific Education Opportunities

Harvard Macy Institute

The Harvard Macy Institute is a collaborative effort of Harvard Medical School, Harvard Graduate School of Education, and Harvard Business School established by a grant from the Josiah Macy Jr. Foundation to drive health education reform and innovation. The institute currently offers three professional development programs targeted at leaders in health education including academic deans, training program directors, and curriculum developers (http://www.harvardmacy.org/Programs/Overview.aspx).

The Program for Educators in Health Professions lists a goal of enhancing the professional development of physicians, basic scientists, and other healthcare professionals as educators through instruction in the five major themes of learning and teaching, curriculum, evaluation, leadership, and information technology. The program enrolls 60 participants to aid in completing an educational project of their own design. Two on-campus sessions are held, 11 days in the winter and 6 days in the spring, during which learners engage in faculty-led small groups for the discussion of the themes and refinement of each scholar's home institution project for educational change.

The Leading Innovations in Health Care and Education Program is designed to enable educational leaders to develop their own action plans for leading and managing change to fulfill their institution's educational mission. Participants completing this program are equipped to strategically lead changes within rapidly evolving healthcare systems and educational programs, known as "disruptive innovation," and pursue a focused institutional innovation project matched with their interests and current institutional needs. This course requires one on-campus session and is conducted in a small group format.

A Systems Approach to Assessment in Health Professions Education is a program designed to allow participants to utilize assessment information in creative ways that allow them to more effectively define their goals, measure performance, and promote their institutional mission. Multiple facets of academic assessment are addressed in the course curriculum, including learning and acquisition of competencies, teaching, education effort and scholarship, program efficacy, and institutional alignment of resources to support the mission of education. This course requires one on-campus workshop conducted in a variety of teaching formats, but each participant is assigned to an institutional planning group to discuss and refine the assessment and evaluation challenges for each individual's institution.

All courses require an electronic application that includes a photo and a one-page biosketch of the applicant's educational activities over the prior 5 years addressing the specific areas of education and professional experience, scholarly interest, and personal background.

Medical Education Research Certificate

Although not intended alone to produce independent medical education researchers, the Medical Education Research Certificate, established by the Group on Educational Affairs of the Association of American Medical Colleges, is a program designed to provide the knowledge necessary to understand the purposes and processes of medical education research, become informed consumers thereof, and become effective collaborators in medical education research (https://www.aamc.org/members/gea/merc).

Program workshops hosted by the AAMC include:

- Data Management and Preparing for Statistical Consultation
- Formulating Research Questions and Designing Studies
- Hypothesis-Driven Research
- Measuring Educational Outcomes with Reliability and Validity

- Introduction to Qualitative Data Collection Methods
- Program Evaluation and Evaluation Research
- Qualitative Analysis Methods in Medical Education
- Questionnaire Design and Survey Research
- Searching and Evaluating the Medical Education Literature
- Scholarly Writing: Publishing Medical Education Research.

Additional workshops may be hosted by other organizations.

The course is designed for clinicians or other educators with a background in medical education but little experience conducting educational research. Completion of six 3-h workshops enables participants to learn research skills enabling collaborative participation in medical education research projects. Registration for the certificate program at the time of press is $100, with an additional $50 for each workshop attended.

Stanford Faculty Development Center for Medical Teachers

The Stanford Faculty Development Center (SFDC) for Medical Teachers offers two courses to academic health center and medical school faculty as training to conduct teaching courses at their home institutions. The center's objectives are to disseminate teaching improvement courses to medical faculty nationally and internationally as well as to provide teaching improvement support to medical teachers at the Stanford campus (http://sfdc.stanford.edu).

Course topics include learning climate, control of session, communication of goals, promotion of understanding and retention, evaluation, feedback, and promotion of self-directed learning. The course targets the principles, guidelines, and behavioral alternatives that teachers can use to improve their effectiveness, and facilitators assert that while the content of the seminars may be discussed during the course, the primary focus is on the process and skills used to teach them. Course organizers believe that teachers at all levels of experience and expertise benefit from review of teaching technique.

Participants begin their training with a 1-month on-site Clinical Teaching facilitator-training course that provides the background knowledge and seminar leadership skills needed to deliver a series of seven 2-h seminars at their home institution. These same faculty may return at a later date for a 5-day course aimed at retraining facilitators to modify and give similar courses to basic science faculty.

International Fellowship in Medical Education

Sponsored by the Foundation for Advancement of International Medical Education and Research, the International Fellowship in Medical Education offers the opportunity to further develop skills in medical education, establish professional communities with other educators around the world, and increase visibility at their home institutions. The program provides individual mentorship for fellows to change medical education in their home countries (http://www.faimer.org/education/ifme/index.html).

The program permits fellows to spend 6–12 months learning aspects of medical education at academic medical centers and medical schools across the United States. Following this experience, fellows may apply for a financial award to pursue a master's degree in health professions education at an approved academic institution. Current participating institutions are Maastricht University in the Netherlands, Stellenbosch University in South Africa, and the University of Illinois at Chicago in the United States.

Essential Skills in Medical Education Course

Aimed at those who would like a greater understanding of the basic principles and best practices of teaching, whether new to the field or holding years of experience, the Essential Skills in Medical Education (ESME) course maintains that all teachers can improve their skills in education (http://www.amee.org/index.asp?lm=140&cookies=True). Sponsored by the Association for Medical Education in Europe (AMEE), the ESME course has been offered since 2005 around the world at various education conferences. It is currently offered in an online format to improve its flexibility in delivery and allow participants to engage with colleagues from around the world.

The course consists of six modules given across 12 weeks that address expectations of health professions educators, learning outcomes and competencies, curriculum development and implementation, principles for effective learning, teaching tool kit, and assessment. Course tuition was listed at 520 British pounds (approximately $825) and includes access to interactive presentations, facilitated online discussion forums, and course materials including a textbook. Dr. Ronald Harden, current editor of the journal Medical Teacher, leads the course.

International Association of Medical Science Educators

The International Association of Medical Science Educators sponsors a Medical Education Fellowship designed in three phases to be completed over a period of 3 years. The program is described as targeted professional development in key aspects of medical education to develop scholars in medical education to enhance and support career advancement (http://iamse.org/fellowship.htm).

The fellowship first begins with completion of the Association for Medical Education in Europe Essential Skills in Medical Education course in the first phase. Phase two entails completion of two 1-day faculty development courses, one at the IAMSE meeting and the other at an additional international meeting. The final phase of the fellowship is completion of an educational scholarship project that demonstrates application of content themes at the participant's home institution. The five content areas fellows are expected to attain proficiency in include curriculum design, teaching methods and strategies, assessment, educational scholarship, and leadership.

Medical science educators who are seeking to become more knowledgeable as educators and leaders are desired applicants for the program. Individuals may also apply following completion of the ESME course. Cost for the fellowship is $550 at time of press and includes required conference workshop modules and materials.

Academy for Innovation in Medical Education Fellowship in Medical Education/Simulation

The University of Ottawa sponsors this program jointly through its Academy for Innovation in Medical Education (AIME) and the University of Ottawa Skills and Simulation Centre (uOSSC). Its overall aim is described as initiating the process of preparing candidates for academic careers as clinician-educators. The program provides specific training and mentorship in curriculum, teaching, and learning as well as in the initiation, design, and conduct of innovative research relevant to the field of health professions education and practice (http://www.med.uottawa.ca/aime/eng/research_fellowship.html).

Fellows will participate in a structured AIME/uOSSC curriculum and other educational activities. Objectives of their fellowship include knowledge of key issues in medical education, adult learning theory, qualitative and quantitative analysis, and educational computer applications. Participation in the development of innovative teaching strategies for continuing education, postgraduate trainees, or undergraduate medical students is highly encouraged. Supervision of a Senior Research Associate and clinical supervisor will be provided for the initiation, design, conduct, and presentation or publication of an educational research project.

Fellows must commit a minimum of 1 year to completion of the program with a minimum of 50 % of protected time away from clinical duty. Enrollment in a master's or doctorate level program in education is strongly recommended to demonstrate a commitment to medical education. The application process varies for those applicants who do and do not plan to engage in clinical work, as those who plan clinical time must first apply and be accepted through the requisite clinical department.

Miscellaneous Programs and Courses

Since faculty development in education has become a major focus in academic surgery, each of the major surgical meetings has devoted time to this topic. The format can vary from breakout sessions (Academic Surgical Congress, Association of

Academic Surgeons) to full-day programs (ACS, APDS, ASE). The focus at each of the meetings can vary, but most are centered on specific topics of interest for educators: enhancing teaching skills, positioning for academic promotion and leadership, and starting research programs. For example, at the ASE, the clerkship directors and coordinators have an all-day course on the basics of running a surgical clerkship and how to troubleshoot common problems. This provides not only a resource for new clerkship directors, but also encourages interaction amongst them since the type of clerkship varies across the country.

Some surgical subspecialties have developed their own mission in education. Due to the evolving training paradigm in cardiothoracic surgery, the Joint Council on Thoracic Surgery Education, Inc. (JCTSE) was formed to specifically improve both surgical resident education and continuing medical education for the practicing cardiothoracic surgeons. Since the "Surgeons as Educators" course by the ACS has been quite popular, enrollment is difficult because of the waiting list and the length of required attendance time. The JCTSE developed a similar but 3-day version of this course entitled "Educate the Educator" (http://www.jctse.org/events.html). With financial support by the major societies in thoracic surgery, surgeons representing each of the training programs are invited to attend the annual course in the summer. Long-term follow-up is also part of the educational mission to develop CT surgical educators at each institution and to help with initiating programs such as simulation and program development.

Simulation-Specific Opportunities

As the realm of simulation in medical education has expanded, the need for individuals with specialized training in the advanced technologies and techniques employed in these centers has grown exponentially. To address this need, several institutions have developed dedicated fellowships to enable clinicians to train in skills and methods necessary to design and implement medical simulation curricula. Some of these opportunities are specific for physicians who have trained in a surgical discipline, while others seek out those with an emergency medicine or anesthesia background, and some will train a physician without a particular specialty designation.

SimPORTAL Simulation Fellowship

This 1-year fellowship at the University of Minnesota seeks to provide a foundation for creating international leaders in the development, evaluation, and delivery of medical education curricula enhanced by simulation technologies (http://www.sim-portal.umn.edu/fellow.htm). Individuals completing this program are expected to be facile in simulation education theory and practice and will participate in curriculum development, research, and enhancement of personal technical skills. Fellows will be involved in simulation classes for medical students and residents, as well as in design and implementation of all surgical simulation activities within SimPORTAL. Simulation research project opportunities will be available via the Center for Research in Education and Simulation Technologies (CREST).

Fellows are expected to attain specific goals in each of the three above domains by the end of their fellowship year. It is anticipated the fellow's curriculum development competency, to which they will devote 40 % of their effort, will entail development of five full simulation curricula, set up and assist in teaching all surgical simulation courses, establish a blueprint for the development of a simulation center at their home institution using ACS criteria, and be an active member of the curriculum and assessment council for SimPORTAL. Publication of at least three papers, design of one simulator, and execution of at least one multicenter validity study will demonstrate research competency, to which 40 % effort will be directed. Twenty percent effort will be directed toward building personal skills, which will include completion of the Fundamentals of Laparoscopic Surgery curriculum and the robotic curriculum.

Applicants to the program must have an M.D. and be enrolled in or have completed a residency in any surgically oriented discipline. International candidates are accepted but must express intent to develop a simulation center and/or program in their home country. Required materials include curriculum vitae, a statement of interest in the fellowship, and letters of recommendation from your current institution and a colleague. Applications are typically due March 15 for a start date of July 1.

Simulation Instructorship Program

This program offered through the center for Simulation Technology and Immersive Learning at Northwestern University provides an opportunity for new graduates from residency programs in the United States to commit to a 2-year faculty position while developing instructional programs in simulation-based medical education across multiple specialties (http://simulation.northwestern.edu/content/education/default.aspx). Instructors are also encouraged to pursue a master's program in an appropriate relevant educational field.

This program began in July 2009 and was led under the visage of Dr. John Vozenilek, a leader in simulation nationally. Instructors engage in the traditional simulation modalities of high-fidelity mannequins and task trainers, in addition to in situ simulation as a teaching tool and a mechanism to improve patient safety. Participants are expected to be clinically active during the time of their appointment, but will also have protected time to attend didactic sessions, participate in research, and teach using immersive technologies. Instructors will also be provided the opportunity to teach workshops at local, regional, and national conferences, develop new curriculum and assessment, contribute to research, and develop their own research program.

Schwartz-Reisman Fellowship in Simulation Medicine

This new program at the Mayo Clinic School of Medicine just accepted its first fellow for a 2-year term beginning July 2012. Fellows in the program will become knowledgeable in simulation-based technologies in the daily operations of the Mayo Clinic Multidisciplinary Simulation Center. The fellowship focuses on training in principles of adult learning theory, advantages and limitations of simulation-based education in health care, simulation typology, and operational techniques of a simulation center (http://www.mayo.edu/multidisciplinary-simulation-center/transformative-education/minnesota/simulation-medicine-fellowship).

Program fellows should expect to advance their skills in the arenas of teaching, group facilitation, grant writing, research, scientific writing, leadership, instructional design, accreditation, budgeting, networking, and management. This will be accomplished through the design and composition of a simulation-based research project, incorporation of simulation-based training into a specialty-specific curriculum, and utilization of simulation courses to optimize patient safety within an established healthcare environment.

Applicants to the Simulation Medicine Fellowship must be college graduates who are pursuing or have already completed an advanced degree and training in academic medicine, including physicians, fellows, residents, nurses, and other advanced allied health personnel. Candidates will undergo background check, drug screening, and health review prior to the start of the fellowship.

Formal Degree in Medical Education

As with other career focuses, those who wish to dedicate their interest to surgical education may wish to pursue a formal degree. Since the needs in medical education differ significantly from other areas of teaching, specific programs have been developed in the form of a master's degree in education for the health professions (MEHP) or master of health profession education (MHPE). These degree programs are generally given as formal classes at a limited number of institutions worldwide. But given the increasing pressure of time and work-related commitments, the wide diversity in professional backgrounds, and the need to design flexible curriculum to fit the needs of the specific individual, there are online courses (e.g., Southern Illinois University, University of Illinois, University of New England) that require only minimal in-class meetings.

Conclusion

As scholarly study of medical education has increasingly attracted top minds across the spectrum of clinical practice, opportunities for individuals to seek out formal training have continued to expand. While it may have once been challenging to find information about such programs, the plethora of opportunities available could result in some scholars having to choose between options. However, this wide array communicates that the academic medicine community has begun to recognize the importance and wide-ranging impact of education on students and trainees in medicine and the benefits conferred by advanced study on this skill set.

Further Reading

1. Glassick CE, Huber MT, Maeroff GI. Scholarship assessed: evaluation of the professoriate. San Francisco: Jossey-Bass; 1997.
2. Sanfey H, Gantt N. Career development resources: academic career in surgical education. Am J Surg. 2012;204(1):126–9.
3. Surgeons as Educators Course. American College of Surgeons. Retrieved 20 Aug 2012, from: http://www.facs.org/education/sre/saeintro.html.
4. ASE Surgical Education Research Fellowship. The Association for Surgical Education. Retrieved 20 Aug 2012, from: http://www.surgicaleducation.com/serf-program.
5. International Scholarships for Surgical Education. American College of Surgeons. Retrieved 20 Aug 2012, from: http://www.facs.org/memberservices/issurged.html.
6. Program overview – enhancing healthcare education through professional development. Harvard Macy Institute. Retrieved 20 Aug 2012, from: http://www.harvardmacy.org/Programs/Overview.aspx.
7. Medical Education Research Certificate Program. Association of American Medical Colleges. Retrieved 20 Aug 2012, from: https://www.aamc.org/members/gea/merc.
8. Stanford Faculty Development Center for Medical Teachers. Stanford University School of Medicine. Retrieved 20 Aug 2012, from: http://sfdc.stanford.edu.
9. International Fellowship in Medical Education. Foundation for Advancement of International Medical Education and Research. Retrieved 20 Aug 2012, from: http://www.faimer.org/education/ifme/index.html.
10. AMEE-ESME Online Course. Association for Medical Education in Europe – An International Association for Medical Education. Retrieved 20 Aug 2012, from: http://www.amee.org/index.asp?lm=140&cookies=True.
11. Medical Educator Fellowship. International Association of Medical Science Educators. Retrieved 20 Aug 2012, from: http://iamse.org/fellowship.htm.
12. AIME/uOSSC Fellowships. University of Ottawa. Retrieved 20 Aug 2012, from: http://www.med.uottawa.ca/aime/eng/research_fellowship.html.
13. SimPORTAL Surgical Simulation Fellowship. University of Minnesota. Retrieved 20 Aug 2012, from: http://www.simportal.umn.edu/fellow.htm.
14. Simulation Technology and Immersive Learning. Northwestern University Feinberg School of Medicine. Retrieved 20 Aug 2012, from: http://simulation.northwestern.edu/content/education/default.aspx.
15. Simulation Medicine Fellowship. Mayo Clinic Multidisciplinary Simulation Center. Retrieved 20 Aug 2012, from: http://www.mayo.edu/multidisciplinary-simulation-center/transformative-education/minnesota/simulation-medicine-fellowship.
16. Joint Council in Thoracic Surgery Education. Educate the Educator Annual Course. http://www.jctse.org/events.html.

Chapter 11
Exploring Advanced Degrees

Jacob A. Greenberg

Introduction

For many years, the majority of surgical residents in academic residency programs across the country have pursued a traditional path towards a career in academic surgery by committing to at least 2 years of research in the basic sciences during their training. While this model continues to be applicable today, the current generation of surgical residents has significantly more options for academic pursuits than their predecessors. Health services, outcomes, translational, and education research have all grown in popularity, and it is increasingly clear that one can be successful in academic surgery by pursuing research in these and a number of other fields. While the skills needed to perform research in the basic sciences can often be learned in the laboratory, the same is not entirely true for health services or education research. Research in these areas requires a different skill set, often employing a mix of both qualitative and quantitative research methods, which are not easily learned outside of a classroom setting. This has led an ever-increasing number of today's residents to pursue additional degrees that may aid in their research efforts. This chapter will explore the role of advanced degrees as they pertain to pursuing a career in education research.

Pros and Cons of Obtaining a Master's or a PhD in Education

The decision to pursue an additional degree is a very personal one and should be in keeping with one's overall career goals. Of all the degrees that can be applied to research in surgical education, either a Master's or a PhD in Education is likely the

J.A. Greenberg, MD, EdM
Department of Surgery,
University of Wisconsin School of Medicine and Public Health,
600 Highland Avenue, K4/728 CSC, Madison, WI 53562, USA
e-mail: greenbergj@surgery.wisc.edu

C.M. Pugh, R.S. Sippel (eds.), *Success in Academic Surgery:*
Developing a Career in Surgical Education, Success in Academic Surgery,
DOI 10.1007/978-1-4471-4691-9_11, © Springer-Verlag London 2013

most beneficial. While most Master's degrees in Education can be earned in a single year, the PhD is more time intensive, often requiring a minimum of a 3-year commitment. While the PhD in Education certainly helps to prepare an individual to become a funded investigator, it comes with a large opportunity cost in terms of lost revenue and time away from the practice of surgery. This may be one of the reasons that most surgeons who choose to pursue an advanced degree opt for the Master's over the PhD.

Pros

Research in education is quite different than other aspects of surgical research. In both basic science and health services/outcomes research, there are a variety of known variables that can usually be controlled for through a variety of techniques. Furthermore the primary end point is normally a well-defined and often quantitative variable that can be calculated and assessed. This is not always the case in education research, where variables are difficult to control for, and the primary end point of learning is extremely challenging to assess quantitatively or qualitatively. While there are many accepted methodologies, such as pre- and posttesting, surveys, interviews, observation, and ethnography, an advanced degree provides the opportunity to study these methodologies as they apply to surgical or other forms of education. Although many of these skills can be acquired through mentoring from an experienced researcher in surgical education, it may be beneficial for some to learn them in a structured didactic setting. Additionally, while it is difficult to know the actual impact of an advanced degree on the perceptions of others, the addition of a Master's or a PhD in Education likely lends some credence to ones' skills as a researcher.

There are other benefits to obtaining an advanced degree in education outside of the research implications. As academic surgeons, teaching both residents and medical students is an integral part of our daily lives. The coursework requirements to earn an advanced degree in education often include some exposure to educational philosophy and teaching methodology, both of which can enrich one's teaching abilities and make them a more effective educator. Additional coursework in curriculum development and curriculum assessment can be useful if one wishes to run a surgical clerkship or residency program. Finally, courses on educational policy and administration can provide a background in educational infrastructure and leadership should one wish to advance through the ranks of a medical school or university.

It is difficult to know the effects that an advanced degree has on one's attractiveness as a candidate for a faculty position. While it certainly may help one obtain their first position, advancement and future positions will be based on academic and clinical productivity rather than the presence or absence of an additional degree.

Cons

While the addition of an advanced degree certainly has some benefits, it is not without its costs. Tuition rates vary between public and private institutions but range anywhere from $10,000 to upwards of $40,000 per year. For a group of people who are often already carrying significant educational debt, the additional year of increased debt and deferred earnings can be quite burdensome. There are multiple societal and institutional grants, scholarships, and fellowship opportunities, such as the Zuckerman Fellowship offered through the Center for Public Leadership at Harvard University, which can help to offset or even negate these costs. However, the extra year of deferred earnings will always be a factor. If one pursues their advanced degree as a resident, he or she may be able to negotiate for tuition funds or salary support from their division or department, but this is obviously institution dependent. Another potential option to control costs is to earn the degree as a part-time student, but this will again lead to a longer time of deferred earnings and may interfere with the timing of residency, practice, or social/family commitments.

Outside of the financial implications of an advanced degree, there is also a significant time commitment associated with earning a Master's or a PhD in Education. Class schedules, assignments, reading, and other activities make it difficult to stay clinically active while pursuing an advanced degree. While this may not be an issue for a resident spending 1 or 2 years in an academic pursuit during their training, it certainly has clinical implications for the practicing surgeon.

One other major factor to consider when selecting a program for an advanced degree is the applicability of the course curriculum to the field of surgery. Most Graduate Schools of Education focus on K–12 and undergraduate education and offer only few courses which pertain to adult education. While courses that focus on qualitative and quantitative research methods as well as curriculum development and assessment should be broadly applicable to a career in surgical education, it is important to also find a program with a strong focus on adult development and principles of adult learning theory. These courses will be more beneficial than those that are structured towards teaching children and adolescents. There are a few institutions that are now offering advanced degrees with a specific focus on surgical education. The Imperial College in London offers a Master's Degree in Surgical Education, and a similar program is offered at the University of Melbourne in Australia. Other programs, such as the Master's of Health Professions Education offered either online or on campus at the University of Illinois Chicago, have less of a surgical focus but are still clearly centered on medical education.

It may also be difficult to maintain a close relationship with one's department and training program during the time away to obtain an advanced degree. While identifying a mentor who focuses on education research within one's program can help to lessen this effect, there is a relative paucity of qualified mentors in education compared to health services researchers and basic scientists. The Surgical Education Research Fellowship offered by the Association for Surgical Education provides

Fellows with the opportunity to work with an established surgical education researcher and is a great option for those without local mentorship. For more information on this program and the overall benefits of mentorship in surgical education, please refer to the Chaps. 9 and 10.

Timing of Obtaining an Advanced Degree

A variety of factors influence the optimal timing for obtaining an advanced degree. From a standpoint of academic productivity, it stands to reason that the sooner one pursues an advanced degree, the greater the impact will be on their career. Having early exposure and grounding in educational research methodology and adult learning theory will help one to devise and complete educational research projects more readily during the early phases of their career. Thus, obtaining the degree during medical school or residency has certain advantages. There are also certain disadvantages in that time away from residency is difficult to come by, tuition is expensive, and the time lag between earning the degree and using it for research may be greater if there is a long period of residency and fellowship in between.

For some, there may be benefits to pursuing the advanced degree later in their training. Interest in educational research may blossom late in residency or as a junior faculty member. While it is difficult to take time away from clinical and academic responsibilities as a practicing surgeon, there are a number of online or offsite options for obtaining a Master's degree. Again, there is no ideal time as everyone's situation will be different, and a variety of factors will influence the optimal timing of obtaining any advanced degree.

Alternative Degrees and the Applicability to Education Research

Beyond advanced degrees in education, there are a variety of other degrees that may be applicable to performing research in surgical education. Degrees with a strong focus on quantitative research methodologies, such as a Master's in Public Health or a Master's in Clinical Investigation or Clinical Epidemiology, can certainly be useful for a career focusing on education research. Additionally, they provide experience in study design, data collection, data analysis, and statistics. There are a wide variety of on-campus and off-campus options to obtain these degrees at many universities across the country. Furthermore, as these degrees may also help one perform health services or outcomes research, they may be funded more readily by surgical divisions or departments.

While these degrees can certainly help one effectively perform a variety of research, they tend to provide less experience in some of the qualitative methodologies that are frequently employed in education research. Additionally, there will not be a focus on other aspects of education that may be pertinent to a career focusing on surgical education. Curriculum development, adult learning theory, educational policy, and evaluations are all part of the activities of surgical educators, and none of these are likely to be learned while obtaining an advanced degree outside of education. Although this knowledge may not be necessary to perform research in surgical education, it will certainly be beneficial for other aspects of one's professional career.

Outside of alternative advanced degrees, there are other options that can help provide one with a background in education research. The Surgical Education Research Fellowship Program offered through the Association for Surgical Education is a 1-year fellowship where each fellow is matched with a mentor from a different institution in order to complete a research project in surgical education. The American College of Surgeons offers an annual "Surgeons as Educators" course which focuses on many aspects of surgical education including curriculum development and performance and program evaluation. These opportunities do not require the larger time commitment of an advanced degree but can certainly help to strengthen one's knowledge and ability to perform research in surgical education.

Conclusion

Ultimately, the decision to pursue an advanced degree in education or an alternative field is a very personal one. While an advanced degree is not necessary to have a productive career focusing on surgical education, some may find it quite beneficial for a variety of reasons. The costs, benefits, opportunity costs, and personal and family factors will all play a role in this decision. Whether or not one chooses to pursue an advanced degree, a career focusing on surgical education can be extremely rewarding and fulfilling.

Further Reading

Capella J, Kasten SJ, Steinemann S, Torbeck L. Guide for research in surgical education. Woodbury: Cine-Med; 2010.
Knowles MS, Holton III EF, Swanson RA. The adult learner. Oxford: Elsevier; 2005.
Searchable list of Graduate School Programs. http://www.gradschools.com/. Accessed on 5 Sep 2013

Chapter 12
Overview of Medical Education Research

Roy Phitayakorn

Background

Medical education research began as a formal field of study in the United States in the 1950s when PhD medical educators were hired to work in the University of Buffalo School of Medicine. As part of an experiment innovatively entitled, "Project in Medical Education," PhD educators offered instruction to medical school faculty in five major medical education domains including the teaching-learning process, the psychosocial nature of medical students, the development of medical education, instructional methods and materials, and the evaluation of effective instruction [1]. One of the results of the Project in Medical Education was the creation of medical education research as a separate discipline within the medical school community. Moreover, it underscored the importance of specific instructional training and evaluation skill sets for medical school faculty. Following this landmark project, many medical schools in the United States hired PhD medical educators to join and enhance their faculty. Therefore, up until the 1990s, medical education researchers were largely individuals with a PhD level background in related disciplines such as cognitive psychology, sociology, and psychometrics [2]. However, the introduction of new medical technologies increased public pressures regarding patient safety, and paradigm shifts in resident education work-hour reforms brought clinical patient care into direct association (and sometimes competition) with medical education research. This connection between education and patient outcomes was coupled with a proliferation of graduate-level medical education training programs for clinical physicians. Indeed, there are currently over 15 master's level programs in medical education in the United States and Canada alone and at least 54 similar programs

R. Phitayakorn, MD, MHPE, (MEd)
Department of Surgery, The Massachusetts General Hospital,
Harvard Medical School, WACC, Suite 460, 15 Parkman Street,
Boston, MA 02114, USA
e-mail: rphitayakorn@partners.org

C.M. Pugh, R.S. Sippel (eds.), *Success in Academic Surgery:*   101
Developing a Career in Surgical Education, Success in Academic Surgery,
DOI 10.1007/978-1-4471-4691-9_12, © Springer-Verlag London 2013

worldwide [3]. Medical education research continued to grow as many medical school promotion and tenure committees rewarded academic physicians with clinician/educator promotion tracks in addition to the traditional clinician/scientist pathways [4]. The net result of all of these changes is that there are now many more medical education researchers who are clinical physicians as opposed to PhDs. This shift creates new challenges as clinical physicians struggle to balance patient care workloads with underfunded medical education projects.

The often conflicting demands of clinical versus research excellence emphasize the need to seek out opportunities to collaborate with PhD level medical education researchers. In fact, the Education Research Committee of the Association for Surgical Education (ERC-ASE) sponsored a workshop at the annual ASE meeting in 2011 and 2012 to address how to maximize the collaborative work between clinical physicians and PhD researchers. This symbiotic relationship ensures that the research projects are theoretically sound and continue to move forward even during busy clinical periods. PhD researchers also benefit from access top clinicians/trainees/students/patients, clinical perspective, training, and skills that would otherwise require completion of a surgical residency to normally acquire. Similar to the rise of interdisciplinary medical disease-based teams, the opportunities for clinical physicians and PhD medical educators to generate high-quality research could never be greater. The next section of this chapter will focus on a few areas of current interest in the surgical education domains of instruction, assessment, and curricular design.

Domain: Instruction and Assessment

Many topics in the research of medical education instruction techniques focus on advances in technology that have created a growing digital-usage gap. Specifically, new computer and mobile communication technologies have resulted in a gap between the so-called digital natives (learners born after 1980) versus digital immigrants (learners born before 1980). Although the true difference between these groups is debatable, the impact of these technological advancements is undeniable. For example, the average member of the millennial generation sends or receives around 60 text messages on a *daily* basis. This profound change in access and utilization of information likely will or already has changed how our trainees proficiently access and assimilate new surgical knowledge. Internet-based surgical curricula with hyperlinks to online surgical textbooks are just the beginning of how surgical educators can maximize knowledge retention and enhance clinical decision-making for both digital natives and late adopters of technology.

Simultaneous with the increase in computer usage and power, surgical technologies are also developing at an ever rapid pace. For example, the explosion of minimally invasive technologies in the late 1980s and early 1990s led to an enormous number of surgical education studies examining different laparoscopic or robotic training curricula and assessment instruments. Many different types of simulators were created or are being created to meet these training demands. Currently developed simulators range from the low-fidelity static models or laparoscopic box trainers to the high-fidelity virtual reality training equipment. Surgical skill simulators appear to benefit most the novice surgical trainee, with less clear advantages to intermediate level learners. Notable challenges with simulation are integrating these simulators into a reduced resident work-hour schedule and the impressive costs of purchasing and maintaining high-fidelity simulators. These challenges disadvantage smaller community-based surgical training programs compared to large academic medical centers. Finally, expert guidance from a surgeon is still ultimately required to ensure correct and adequate skill acquisition for most laparoscopic or robotic tasks. However, few medical centers have worked out satisfactory compensation plans for surgeons who teach residents in the simulation lab versus the operating room.

Future studies will likely adopt a more practical "cost per skill gained" method of evaluation to determine which skills are worth the expense of high-fidelity simulation with expert guidance and which skills can be developed independently with lower cost models of instruction. There are also a growing number of studies that examine not only surgical skill acquisition but how those skills should ultimately be combined with surgical judgment to create a complete operation instead of isolated tasks. Lastly, there are a growing number of studies in the surgical education literature that use spaced simulation sessions to teach surgical skills such as interprofessional teamwork, communication, and professionalism. The development of these nonmanual dexterity-based skills is likely enhanced in the low clinical risk environment that simulation can create and foster. These studies also highlight the importance of future surgical faculty leadership development and the challenges in teaching and debriefing medical students, residents, and surgical peers.

In terms of assessment, surgical educators have just scratched the surface of creating surgical instruments that are both highly valid and reliable. For the resident level of training, the Accreditation Council for Graduate Medical Education (ACGME) and the Resident Review Committee are currently beta testing the new General Surgery Milestones Project. The original ACGME Core Competencies were a largely quantitative program and trainee assessment of whether or not processes were in place to instruct and evaluate for each of the six core competencies (patient care, medical knowledge/skills, practice-based learning and improvement, interpersonal and communication skills, professionalism, and systems-based practice). The Milestones Project is a much more qualitative assessment instrument that examines every trainee and asks questions that highlight what are competent resident behaviors in professionalism, for example. Although the true downstream effects of this project are unclear, the subtext would suggest that trainees who achieved all of the milestones early would be allowed to finish residency training ahead of trainees with deficient milestones. The possible shift from the traditional surgical time-based promotion system to a competency-based system would generate many repercussive research efforts in high-stakes surgical skills assessments, remediation of poorly performing trainees or colleagues, and enhanced integration of board certification with actual clinical outcomes. It is inevitable that further research will be stimulated in determining maintenance of certification for attending surgeons, the acquisition of new surgical skills, and the assessment of lifelong professional development.

Domain: Curricula Development

Many surgical educators get their first taste for education research when they are asked to revise or create a surgical curriculum. Unfortunately, as discussed in Chap. 15 of this book, curriculum development is often not held to the same standards as experimental studies and curricula can be difficult to publish – which may be an important promotional/tenure criterion. However, the need for scholarship with curricula development has never been greater as there is an increasing amount of information in each surgical discipline to be learned by an average surgical trainee.

For example, in general surgery alone, there are hundreds of textbooks that cover the different disciplines included in general surgery such as endocrine surgery, trauma/urgent care surgery, cardiac surgery, thoracic surgery, transplant, colorectal surgery, vascular surgery, pediatric surgery, surgical oncology, plastic surgery, breast surgery, surgical critical care, and burn surgery. The Surgical Council on Resident Education (SCORE) general surgery curriculum was an important first step towards gaining consensus on the patient care, medical knowledge, and surgical procedures that were essential for a general surgery resident to demonstrate proficiency upon completion of the residency. The SCORE curriculum divides the ACGME core competency of patient care into 28 organ-based patient care categories of around 700 topics (subdivided into focused and broad) and 304 operations (subdivided into essential-common, essential-uncommon, and complex). Similarly, the SCORE curriculum also divides the medical knowledge core competency into 13 categories of around 78 topics. Future curricula research will likely focus on which aspects of the curricula are most needed for a general surgeon and most importantly how and why do curricula coupled with valid and reliable assessment impact daily patient care.

High-Quality/High-Impact Medical Education Research

Several studies have suggested that there is a lack of scientific rigor in many medical education studies. This finding can be detrimental to the progress of the field of medical education and may undermine a medical education researcher's ability to seek competitive institutional funding and credibility among their peers. Cook et al. [5] reviewed 105 medical education articles published in well-known peer-reviewed medical education journals from 2003 to 2004. They found that only 16 % of the articles had a clearly defined study design and less than half of the articles had operationally defined independent and dependent variables (47 and 32 %, respectively). Even more alarming was that only 42 % of studies reported Institutional

Review Board approval and/or a participant consent process. These results should not discourage someone interested in conducting surgical education research, but rather emphasize the great need for high-quality education studies. To avoid these pitfalls, the rest of this chapter will focus on key questions that should be considered when planning a successful surgical education research project.

Question #1: What Is Already Known About the Topic?

Many surgeons mistakenly assume that only surgical journals contain articles pertinent to their research interests when starting with a literature review. However, it is important to think broadly at this research step and think of disciplines outside of surgery and even medicine itself that may glean useful insights into the research problem/question. These disciplines include cognitive science/psychology, behavioral science, human factors, computer science/engineering, education/counseling, neuroscience, sociology/anthropology, military, business, and the performing arts to name a few. For example, if a surgeon was interested in how interprofessional teams perform in the operating room, a literature review could include other high-stakes/high-performance teams such as medical evacuation flight teams, wildfire firefighters, or nuclear power plant workers. A reference librarian is an invaluable resource at this step and can help ensure an adequate sampling of the available literature. The ultimate goal of a thorough literature review is to create the beginnings of a theoretical framework to understand how the research fits into the larger fabric of what is already known.

Question #2: What Is/Are the Purpose and Research Question(s) of This Study?

This question addresses the purpose of the study. Unfortunately, many medical education studies simply describe how a project was done, but do not address why the project was started in the first place. Researchers must step back and clearly articulate the research questions and hypotheses. This is vital not only for communicating the innovation and results of one's work but will also allow for efficient use of resources. Just as in the basic sciences, the research questions should include the study population, the intervention (independent variable), the outcome (dependent variable), and the relationship between the variables. As an example, a hypothetical medical education research question could be, "Does problem-based learning in a surgical clerkship improve medical students' teamwork skills?" In this example, the study population is medical students, the intervention is problem-based learning, the outcome is teamwork skills, and the relationship is improvement. Good research questions contribute to the medical education literature and will strengthen the theoretical framework created in Question #1 above.

Question #3: What Is the Optimal Study Design?

Chapter 13 will discuss in detail the multitude of options in selecting a study design. This question is essential as many medical education studies are weakened by flawed study designs that are not reproducible and generate poorly generalizable results. It is important to consult with experienced medical education researchers at this point to evaluate the proposed study design. Local expertise may also be found by doing a PubMed (www.pubmed.com) or Google Scholar (www.scholar.google. com) search with your topic and institution or city. Surgeons with a basic science background may feel overwhelmed at this point in the development process as they have created complex National Institutes of Health 5-year type study designs. A more realistic starting point is a pilot-type project that focuses on either the researcher's home institution or a few neighboring ones where the researcher has contacts. Splitting large research questions into more manageable pilot-sized studies allows regular progress to occur along a research pathway and also prevents researcher burnout or loss of interest.

Question #4: Does the Research Project Need Approval from the Local Institutional Review Board?

Unfortunately, there is little guidance at the national level about what types of medical education projects warrant exempt versus expedited versus full review by the local Institutional Review Board (IRB). This issue is particularly problematic for multi-institutional education research projects where the study may be exempt at one institution but requires a full rereview at another institution. In general, all medical education projects should be submitted to the local IRB for review. If one is unsure about the type of review for a given medical education project, it is best to contact a member of the IRB *prior* to submitting the paperwork. The IRB members frequently welcome the chance to talk about the project in advance which prevents unnecessary review and wasted effort.

Summary

From very modest beginnings in a single department of a single institution, medical education research has slowly transformed into a tenurable/promotable specialty of medicine in medical centers across the world. This growth will likely accelerate in the future as a direct result of many exciting and challenging issues in the domains of instruction, assessment, and curriculum development. A major threat to the progress of medical education research is the allocation of scarce funding mechanisms and the historical reporting of observational/descriptive studies with unclear research questions or goals. Recognition and prevention of these deficiencies will ensure that medical education research continues to advance for the enhancement of our trainees and ultimately improve overall patient care and delivery.

References

1. Hitchcock MA. Introducing professional educators into academic medicine: stories of exemplars. Adv Health Sci Educ Theory Pract. 2002;7(3):211–21.
2. Norman G. Fifty years of medical education research: waves of migration. Med Educ. 2011;45(8):785–91.
3. Tekian A, Harris I. Preparing health professions education leaders worldwide: a description of masters-level programs. Med Teach. 2012;34(1):52–8.
4. Glick TH. How best to evaluate clinician-educators and teachers for promotion? Acad Med. 2002;77(5):392–7.
5. Cook DA, Beckman TJ, Bordage G. Quality of reporting of experimental studies in medical education: a systematic review. Med Educ. 2007;41(8):737–45.

Chapter 13
Promoting Excellence in Surgical Educational Research

Sara Kim, Sinan Jabori, and Carlos A. Pellegrini

Background

Welcome to the world of educational research. You may already have prior experiences in designing and conducting research studies or you may be seeking new ways to teach and assess your trainees by exploring educational studies reported in surgical journals. Regardless of your prior exposure to research, it is critical to understand the building blocks of how to design a good research study. This chapter introduces you to the basic concepts of educational research using actual examples from published studies in surgical education.

The domain of surgical education offers rich opportunities to develop, test, and implement novel teaching and evaluation methods in order to improve the quality of education targeting students, residents, and practicing surgeons. Designing and conducting rigorous educational research studies is essential so that the results you report are scientifically credible. At the heart of research is the application of research findings to other educational settings and subjects. We call this application generalizability. For example, a curriculum designed to improve residents' technical

S. Kim, PhD (✉)
Department of Surgery, Institute of Simulation and Interprofessional Studies (ISIS),
School of Medicine, University of Washington,
356410, Seattle, WA 98195, USA
e-mail: sarakim@uw.edu

S. Jabori
Division of Vascular Surgery, UCLA Gonda (Goldschmied) Vascular Center,
David Geffen School of Medicine at UCLA,
200 Medical Plaza, 5th floor, Los Angeles, CA, USA
e-mail: sjabori@mednet.ucla.edu

C.A. Pellegrini, MD, FACS, FRCSI (Hon.)
Department of Surgery, School of Medicine, University of Washington,
356410, Seattle, WA 98195, USA
e-mail: pellegri@u.washington.edu

C.M. Pugh, R.S. Sippel (eds.), *Success in Academic Surgery:*
Developing a Career in Surgical Education, Success in Academic Surgery,
DOI 10.1007/978-1-4471-4691-9_13, © Springer-Verlag London 2013

proficiencies can be applied to medical students on the following condition: the research study you conduct to examine whether the curriculum is effective needs to be grounded in the basic principles of research. The level of rigor in research ensures generalizability. There are a number of factors that threaten generalizability, such as an insufficient number of study subjects or unreliable data collection instruments. This chapter focuses on specific aspects of research design so that you can maximize your ability to generalize findings to other educational context and trainees. We will first begin with an overview of research design followed by explanations of the core concepts in the context of published surgical educational studies.

Overview of Research Design

The main methodologies in educational research can be largely divided into *quantitative* and *qualitative* study design depending on how data were collected, analyzed, and reported. A mixed study design, which is not covered in this chapter, combines both quantitative and qualitative data collection and analytical methods. The following five questions can serve a useful purpose in understanding the key differences between the quantitative and qualitative research design methods:

1. What is the main purpose of the research being conducted?
2. How is the size of research subjects determined?
3. What are the key methods for collecting data from research subjects?
4. How are research data analyzed?
5. How are research data reported?

Let us examine each question in detail below.

What Is the Main Purpose of Research Being Conducted?

In quantitative study design, the main research goal is to test research hypotheses. Hypotheses are typically determined a priori or in advance. Key research findings are interpreted based on whether hypotheses are confirmed or rejected. For example, let us assume you designed a new surgical skill curriculum in your residency program and are interested in exploring whether it actually improves your residents' skills. Your hypothesis may be that the new curriculum improves residents' technical proficiencies compared to the old curriculum. If your findings show a higher proficiency level in residents' skills after implementing the new curriculum and compared to the old, you can then accept your hypothesis as true.

On the other hand, the key focus of qualitative research design is not typically about testing a research hypothesis that was predetermined. Rather, its focus is to build a theory or a conceptual framework that explains a phenomenon or behavioral trends. This is achieved through an inductive approach by analyzing the collected data from subjects, identifying recurrent themes, and proposing a conceptual framework.

The most widely used theory-building method is the "grounded theory," which examines the meanings of relations and patterns in information collected from research subjects. We will later see an excellent example of a qualitative research study.

How Is the Size of Research Subjects Determined?

In quantitative research studies, generalizability of findings to other educational settings hinges on two factors: (a) how research subjects are sampled and (b) whether your study is powered by a sufficient number of subjects in the study. If you are testing the effectiveness of a new suturing skill curriculum, drawing your subjects from multiple surgical fields including surgery, obstetrics/gynecology, and otolaryngology would allow you to apply your findings to a larger population representing these selected fields. The other factor that affects generalizability is the number of research subjects. How do you determine up front how many subjects you may need in your study? The answer lies in a "power analysis," which will be discussed in detail later. For now, it is sufficient for you to understand that there are statistical methods to help determine the number of subjects to recruit, and these methods ensure that the results you find are not based on chance but are statistically valid. When a research study includes a power analysis, it lends a credible foundation to how results can be interpreted. Having said this, you may be constrained by a fixed number of subjects, such as the number of residents in your program. This is where multi-specialty or multi-institutional research design can help strengthen the power of your study, therefore, the generalizability of research findings.

Unlike what happens in quantitative research, where the number of subjects sampled for the study bolsters or weakens the degree to which findings can be generalized to a larger population, qualitative research frequently relies on "purposeful" or "convenience" sampling when recruiting study subjects. An equivalent statistical method, such as a power analysis, to determine the number of subjects is not available in qualitative study design. Instead, it is important to remember a concept, *saturation*, which is at the core of qualitative analyses. Research subjects are recruited until researchers exhaust or saturate possible patterns and trends in data without prematurely terminating the recruitment of subjects or data analysis processes. This means if an insufficient number of subjects are recruited, the scope and depth of information that researchers set out to report can be compromised.

What Are the Key Methods for Collecting Data from Research Subjects?

The method of collecting data in a quantitative study depends on the type and number of *independent variables* (e.g., age, ethnicity, practice settings) and *dependent or outcomes variables* (e.g., knowledge, attitudes, perceptions, or behaviors). Researchers rely on multiple methods for collecting data in quantitative studies: tests for assessing knowledge (e.g., multiple-choice, open-ended questions), checklists/ global ratings for assessing technical skills (e.g., OSATS – Objective Structured Assessment of Technical Skills), surveys or questionnaires for examining attitudes or collecting demographic information, computer-generated data from simulators that monitor trainees' technical proficiencies (e.g., LapSim – laparoscopic surgical simulator), or motion-tracking devices for measuring subjects' procedural efficiencies. These methods yield data that can be quantified to show improvements or trends of target outcomes. It is critical that researchers pilot their data collection instruments with content experts or with subjects comparable to the actual research subjects, particularly if the instruments were not previously established to be reliable or valid. Later in this chapter, we will discuss, in more detail, implications of using unreliable measurements and how generalizability can be compromised as a result.

In contrast to quantitative studies, qualitative researchers collect data from subjects through focus groups with multiple individuals or one-on-one interviews using predetermined sets of questions. It is critical that researchers pilot interview questions to ensure that the questions posed to research subjects would not create an unwanted bias and instead, generate rich layers of content for analyses. Typically, focus group or interview sessions are audio- or videotaped for analyzing the content. The tapes represent your raw data, which then must be analyzed.

How Are Research Data Analyzed?

Researchers typically analyze their quantitative data using statistical software programs. SPSS (Statistical Package for the Social Sciences) and SAS (Statistical Analysis System) are common programs. It is important to know two critical points when handling datasets. First, you have to choose the right analytical methods depending on the research questions you are posing. To put it simply, if you have one participant group and one dependent variable (e.g., level of trainees' skills), you will typically report descriptive statistics including frequency counts, mean scores, and standard deviations (i.e., distributions of scores from the mean). If you have two variables (e.g., level of skills, time on task), you may report correlations between the two. Analyzing two or more independent variables (e.g., level of training, gender, years of experience, number of practice hours) and dependent variables (e.g., economy of motion, time to completion) involves advanced analytical methods, called multivariate analyses (e.g., multiple regressions).

After choosing the analytical methods, researchers need to demonstrate that the key results they find have statistical significance. Statistical significance is expressed as $p < 0.05$ or $p < 0.01$ to denote the level of probability (i.e., 95 % or 99 %) that researchers choose to use for accepting or rejecting their hypotheses. For example, let us say subjects in Group A (treatment group) complete a new curriculum to improve their teamwork skills while subjects in Group B (control group) are not exposed to the same curriculum. Then, you provide identical teamwork scenarios to subjects in both groups and rate their performances using a checklist. Your analysis should demonstrate that differences in scores observed between the two groups were not based on chance, but rather there existed real differences between the two groups. The best way to show these real differences is by including the actual differences in means, confidence intervals, and p-values associated with the statistical tests you conducted. We will discuss later some of the tests that are used to establish statistical significance when we review published research studies.

As mentioned earlier, the key to data analysis in qualitative studies is saturation. The goal of qualitative researchers is to examine all possible patterns, relations, and meanings of information collected from focus group and interview subjects. Typically, more than one researcher analyzes transcribed content from focus groups and interviews to examine themes that arise from the transcript and develop thematic codes to cluster verbal information into categories. In addition to coding the transcripts manually, researchers may also use content analysis software programs, such as ATLAS.ti (Archive for Technology, the Life World, and Everyday Language) or NUD*IST (Non-numerical Unstructured Data Indexing, Searching, and Theorizing). The process involved in analyzing qualitative data can be very time and labor intensive as researchers engage in multiple, iterative discussions and consensus building until they are satisfied that all possible thematic codes are identified from the transcripts. Because of this labor-intensive nature of data analyses, most studies report findings based on a small number of subjects. You may be wondering whether this creates a threat to generalizability of qualitative findings to a larger population. You are right! This is one limitation of qualitative study design. However, the key contribution of qualitative studies is to develop a theoretical or conceptual framework to understand a phenomenon or to explore an issue in depth, such as implications of resident burnout on patient care or medical students' career interests in surgery.

How Are Research Data Reported?

Quantitative results are usually presented in graphs, charts, and tables to illustrate trends over time, comparative differences in subjects who undergo study treatments (i.e., exposure to a new curriculum vs. no exposure), or a cross-sectional view of data. In contrast, qualitative researchers may use diagrams or charts to illustrate how their findings inform a theoretical framework. Frequently, qualitative studies report key thematic codes and include subjects' verbatim or paraphrased quotes as examples to illustrate the meanings of thematic codes.

We just completed a big picture survey of quantitative and qualitative research design. The most important points for you to remember are summarized in Table 13.1.

Table 13.1 An overview of research study design

Research design/questions	Quantitative research design	Qualitative research design
1. What is the main purpose of the research being conducted?	To confirm or reject research hypotheses	To build a theory of a phenomenon or behaviors of subjects
2. How is the number of the research subjects determined?	A statistical technique called power analysis can help determine up front how many subjects are needed	Convenience or purposeful sampling until saturation of themes is attained
3. What are the key methods for collecting data from research subjects?	Assessment instruments that yield quantitative data about subjects' behaviors or attitudes, such as multiple-choice questions, survey, checklists	Focus groups or interviews with subjects using interview questions
4. How are research data analyzed?	Use of statistical software programs to analyze relationship between independent and dependent variables	Content analysis for identifying emerging themes. Software programs are also available for examining interrelationship among thematic codes
5. How are research data reported?	Tables, graphs, charts	Diagrams and quotes from study participants

Understanding Research Methodologies Using Published Studies

Now let us move to specific aspects of research design using two examples of published studies in surgical education. One study by Immenroth et al. [3] represents a quantitative research study focusing on the impact of mental training on technical proficiencies. The second study by Musselman et al. [10] is a qualitative research study that examines how residents and practicing surgeons perceive intimidation and harassment during surgical training. These two studies represent many aspects of research methodologies and serve to help you understand basic concepts in an actual research context.

Example 1: Quantitative Research Study

Box 13.1 provides a synopsis of a quantitative research study published in *Annals in Surgery* by Immenroth and colleagues [3]. It focuses on an interesting educational technique involving mental training to help surgeons improve their technical skills. Mental training uses visualization and internal verbalization of procedural steps so that surgeons develop a mental picture of the procedure in preparation for an actual procedure. Now let us analyze this study using the five research design questions we discussed before.

Box 13.1 Example 1: Research Study Using Quantitative Research Methodologies

Objective

The objective of this research is to examine the effectiveness of mental training on the performance of laparoscopic cholecystectomy. Mental training is a technique involving systematic and repeated visualizing and verbalizing of procedural movements.

Methods

1. Study design: A *randomized-controlled trial*.
2. Subjects: A total of 98 surgeons attending training courses on basic laparoscopy offered by the European Surgical Institute, Norderstedt, Germany. The authors report that at least 90 participants would provide sufficient *power* (80 %) to detect an intergroup difference at a significance level of 5 %.
3. Intervention: All participants completed a 2-day mental training course. Following the baseline performance assessment, participants were *randomly assigned* to three study conditions: (a) no additional training (control, $n=35$), (b) additional practical training ($n=32$), and (c) additional mental training involving a 90-min one-to-one tutorial ($n=31$).
4. Performance assessment: A *baseline* and *follow-up* performance of laparoscopic cholecystectomy was assessed using a Pelvi-Trainer simulator. Videotapes of performance were rated by four *evaluators,* who assessed performance based on a *modified OSATS (Objective Structured Assessment of Technical Skills)* including 11 checklist items and five global rating items.
5. Data analysis: Baseline and follow-up performance differences across three groups were analyzed using *analysis of variance (ANOVA)*. Subsequent pairwise comparisons were made based on *t-tests*.

Results

When comparing the baseline and follow-up performance based on the OSATS checklist, statistical significances were found between mental and practical training groups ($p=0.024$) as well as between mental training and control groups ($p=0.040$). Thus, participants undergoing additional mental training achieved a greater improvement at follow-up compared to other groups.

Source: Immenroth et al. [2].

What Is the Purpose of the Research Being Conducted?

The purpose of this study is to examine whether additional mental training has a positive effect on surgeons' performance of laparoscopic cholecystectomy. So the main research hypothesis is that surgeons who receive additional mental training will demonstrate a superior technical proficiency in laparoscopic cholecystectomy compared to surgeons who do not undergo additional mental training. A research hypothesis is often stated in a format that allows researchers to accept or reject it. The main research design in the study by Immenroth and colleagues is a randomized controlled trial (RCT) for testing their hypothesis. RCTs are considered to be the gold standard of quantitative studies. They involve randomly assigning subjects to study groups so that possible biases, both systematic and random, can be avoided in favor of a particular subject group (i.e., Group A includes mostly female subjects and Group B mostly males, creating a gender bias). In this study, the authors created three study groups and randomly assigned subjects to a group that received no additional training (35 subjects), a group that received additional practical training (32 subjects), and a group that received additional mental training (31 subjects) following a basic training session that all study participants completed.

How Is the Size of the Research Subjects Determined?

The authors report that 98 surgeons attending basic laparoscopy training courses participated in the study. For an educational study, this is a fairly large subject sample. The authors report a power analysis as a justification for the size of the subjects in their study. As discussed earlier in the overview section, power is defined as the likelihood to detect an effect of a study intervention (i.e., a new curriculum), if indeed an effect exists. Traditionally, the minimum power is set at 0.80. In the current study, the authors report that at least 90 participants would provide sufficient *power* (80 %) to detect an intergroup difference at a significance level of 5 % (or $p < 0.05$). This means the study is adequately powered by the subject size and, furthermore, if the authors find differences in performance among subjects across the three study groups, that differences would not be by chance alone. For readers who are interested in more advanced pointers, Box 13.2 below provides a detailed guideline on how to conduct a power analysis.

Box 13.2 A Guideline for Conducting a Power Analysis

When recruiting subjects to control and intervention groups, an online tool, such as G*Power 3 (http://www.psycho.uni-duesseldorf.de/abteilungen/aap/gpower3/download-and-register), can guide researchers' study design. To determine a sample size, researchers would typically need to know up front three data elements: (1) What is the *significance level* of "p" value I am targeting (i.e., $p < 0.05$, $p < 0.01$)?; (2) what is the projected *effect size*[a] in my study based on prior published studies (i.e., 0.3 = small effect, 0.5 = medium effect, 0.7 = large effect)?; and (3) what is the level of *power* I am aiming for (i.e., the likelihood that I am correctly rejecting the null hypothesis)? In a simplified, hypothetical randomized controlled study involving two groups of subjects, a researcher would select in G*Power 3, *t-tests* for comparison of means between two independent groups and enter a *p-value* of 0.05, *effect size* of 0.5, and a *power* of 0.80 to obtain a total sample size of 102 (51 in control, 51 in intervention). This would translate as follows: A sample size of 102 would be required to obtain a power of 0.80 in detecting a moderate effect size of 0.5 (at $p = 0.05$). It may be helpful to know that there is an inverse relationship between anticipated effect size and sample size when one wants to maintain an acceptable power. That is, it takes a larger sample to detect a small effect and smaller sample to detect a large effect.

[a] Effect size is commonly referred to as Cohen's d and is derived by calculating the differences in mean scores of two study groups and dividing them by a pooled standard deviation.

What Are the Key Methods for Collecting Data from Research Subjects?

The authors report that they modified an existing technical skills rating tool, OSATS (Objective Structured Assessment of Technical Skills), which included 11 checklist items and five global rating items to assess surgeons' technical skills in laparoscopic cholecystectomy. The former is used to record the presence or absence of a targeted behavior in trainees (e.g., explored the liver, exposed the cystic duct and the cystic artery). The latter is used for a holistic assessment of overall technical skills based on a scale of 1 (very poor) to 5 (very good). Typically, an evaluator or multiple evaluators rate performances while they observe subjects completing tasks in real time or while watching videotaped sessions. OSATS was previously created and tested for its psychometric rigor; therefore, it is a *reliable* and *valid* assessment measure. Immenroth and colleagues used this existing reliable and valid assessment tool, which makes their data collection scientifically sound. Had they developed an assessment tool in-house instead, they would have to establish and report its reliability and validity.

These two concepts, reliability and validity, are at the heart of assessment. What is the significance of reliability? When a flawed assessment tool or process is used to generate data, researchers' ability to apply the findings to comparable population groups is seriously compromised. For example, an unreliable assessment tool may include inaccurate items, excessively difficult items, or items that create a bias against certain population groups. Furthermore, when only one evaluator observes a learner's performance, that evaluator may introduce biases that could distort research findings. For readers interested in learning more about different ways to establish reliability, please see Box 13.3.

Validity defines whether scores generated from an assessment instrument measure what they intend to measure. For example, you create an observation rating form to assess team communication skills. How do you ensure that the items in the form actually measure team communication? Box 13.4 describes four ways to establish validity. If you want to skip this detail, simply remember that without validity evidence, findings you report may raise questions in terms of their scientific rigor.

Box 13.3 Types of Reliability

Typically, there are four types of reliability a researcher can report: (1) test-retest reliability, (2) inter-rater reliability, (3) internal consistency, and (4) G-study. *Test-retest reliability* is calculated by correlating scores from a test taken more than once by subjects who are drawn from homogenous groups (i.e., PGY1 cohort). A high reliability ($r = 0.80$) points to the robustness of tests when administered multiple times to comparable groups of test takers. *Inter-rater reliability* measures the degree to which raters agree on their assessment of learners' performance. The reliability can be derived simply by averaging the percentage of agreement between two raters or by using a more advanced measure, such as Kappa statistics, when establishing reliability among multiple raters. *Internal consistency*, frequently expressed as Cronbach's alpha (0–1.00), measures the degree to which test items correlate with one another, which signifies how well items measure the target "construct" or assessment domain, such as critical thinking skills. A low level of Cronbach's alpha suggests the test is unreliable in measuring the learning domain that test developers intend to target. Cronbach's alpha internal consistency treats possible measurement errors, whether they involve subjects, test items, or test environment, as random and undifferentiated. When examining multiple sources of both systematic and unsystematic measurement error is of interest, researchers can rely on a method called *Generalizability Study* (G-Study). The G-Study analytical model can simultaneously account for sources of variation and error in subjects, test occasion (pre-, post-, delayed test), and the interaction between subjects and occasion. A software program to conduct G-Studies can be freely downloaded from http://www.education.uiowa.edu/centers/casma/computer-programs.aspx#genova.

Box 13.4 Types of Validity

Validity types are largely categorized into the following: (1) content validity, (2) construct validity, (3) concurrent validity, and (4) predictive validity. *Content validity*, which is widely reported in research studies, represents the weakest form of validity. It frequently involves a panel of experts recruited by researchers, who review the content of data collection instruments for quality assurance. *Content validity* is provided in descriptive terms such as "Content experts reviewed the assessment instrument and provided feedback to improve its quality." *Construct validity* demonstrates differentiations in performance by subjects recruited from different training levels, such as experts, intermediate trainees, and novices. When researchers find that assessment instruments yield the highest scores for experts and the lowest scores for novices after subjects complete identical tasks, the construct validity is established. *Concurrent validity* measures whether performance on a test that is newly constructed correlates with performance on an established test that covers a similar content domain. Reporting the concurrent validity provides one level of evidence that the new test is valid in its measurement rigor. *Predictive validity* involves measuring performance in one study setting and correlating it to performance in another setting. Using OSATS for assessing residents' skills as an example, when performance on a task trainer in a simulation center correlates with performance in the operating room and that correlation is statistically significant; researchers conclude that scores generated from OSATS have a predictive validity.

It is worth noting that the mainstream educational thinking outside of medical education promotes the view that construct validity encompasses all sources of validity evidence. For more information, please see Downing [1].

How Are Research Data Analyzed?

In the study by Immenroth et al., data from subjects in the three study groups were collected prior to and following training sessions. These two data points (baseline and follow-up) from three study groups are entered into a statistical software program and examined as to whether there were differences in performance improvements across the three groups and whether these differences were statistically significant. The authors report that they performed an ANOVA, which stands for one-way analysis of variance. ANOVA is used for comparing scores from at least two study groups or more. When a study includes one or two study groups, t-tests are used to examine whether mean scores (i.e., pretest, posttest) within a group or between two groups are statistically significant. When conducting an ANOVA, what you are detecting is whether there is an overall statistical significance in scores across study groups. As the authors reported, a subsequent statistical test, such as a t-test, helps pinpoint where the differences actually occurred between study groups (i.e., between no additional training and additional mental training, between additional practical training and additional mental training, between no additional training and additional practical training).

How Are Research Data Reported?

If you read the entire article, the authors first reported that the ANOVA resulted in an overall statistically significant difference in the scores across the three study groups. The authors subsequently report that they found a statistical difference based on t-tests between mental and practical training groups and this difference had a less than 3 % probability ($p=0.024$) of happening by chance. Similarly, there was a difference between the mental training and control group (no training) with a less than 5 % probability ($p=0.040$) of this difference occurring as a result of chance. Based on this key result, the researchers accepted their hypothesis that additional mental training led to improved performance by subjects who received additional mental training compared to those who did not.

Example 2: Qualitative Research Study

Now let us turn to a very different research study that is based on qualitative research methods. The study by Musselman et al. [10], which is published in *Medical Education*, is summarized in Box 13.5.

Box 13.5 Example 2: Research Study Using Qualitative Research Methodologies

Objective

The study focuses on developing *a grounded theory* of (a) how perceived meanings of intimidation and harassment are constructed by staff surgeons and surgical residents and (b) how intimidation and harassment impact the learning environment and socialization of surgical trainees.

Methods

1. Study design: Qualitative design based on *group interviews* and *semi-structured interviews* with video vignettes as discussion triggers.
2. Subjects: *Convenience* and *purposeful sampling* of 36 subjects (22 staff surgeons, 14 residents), who participated in one of 5 group interviews (3 staff groups and 2 resident groups) and 22 individual interviews (14 staff and 8 residents) conducted at two academic centers.
3. Data collection and analyses: Interviews were audiotaped. Three reviewers (a surgical resident, an operating room nurse, and a qualitative researcher) engaged in ***iterative and recursive reading*** of transcripts and generated *categories of emergent themes*. Through an iterative consensus-building process, the reviewers agreed upon the final categorization of themes. The NVivo qualitative data analysis software was used to examine interrelationships among *thematic categories*.

Results

Interviewees offered rationalization of behaviors that are perceived as intimidation and harassment: (a) If an acceptable educational purpose is found, a behavior may not be perceived as intimidation and harassment; (b) there are positive pedagogical and clinical roles that justify a behavior that is perceived as intimidation and harassment; and (c) necessary actions, particularly for ensuring patient safety, may legitimize behaviors perceived as intimidation and harassment.

Source: Musselman et al. [3].

What Is the Main Purpose of the Research Being Conducted?

Musselman et al. addresses a topic of intimidation and harassment as perceived by surgical residents and attendings. Instead of designing a survey to collect perceptions of these study subjects that can be reported in a quantifiable manner, the authors chose to conduct qualitative research design for the purpose of explaining these perceptions in depth based on direct interactions with surgeons and residents.

How Is the Size of Research Subjects Determined?

The size of the subject pool is determined by convenience and purposeful sampling as the authors reported. Subjects were recruited from departments of surgery at two academic centers (i.e., convenience sampling). The authors relied on purposeful sampling of subjects as well, which means, "Sampling was completed when no new concepts related to the research questions were discovered" (p. 928). Therefore, subject recruitment and data analyses go hand in hand in qualitative research studies.

What Are the Key Methods for Collecting Data from Research Subjects?

The authors report that they collected data using two methodologies: (a) focus groups with multiple subjects and (b) individual interviews, both of which were audiotaped. In the full article, the authors describe pros and cons with each data collection method. Focus groups largely depend on group dynamics among participants. This creates a positive effect where participants' stories can serve as triggers that draw out complementary or contradictory perspectives of participants. On the other hand, dominant participants can possibly overshadow other participants, who may not feel safe to openly discuss sensitive topics, such as intimidation and harassment. Individual interviews create a sense of safety for participants, but it can be both time and labor intensive as researchers need to conduct multiple interviews before sufficient information is collected from research participants. In the study by Musselman et al., they structured individual interviews using open-ended questions to elicit participants' understanding of intimidation and harassment. Also, in order to shape and direct the scope of interview sessions, researchers used video vignettes of scenarios that portrayed instances of intimidation and harassment using simulated interactions between surgeons and residents. These video vignettes served a useful purpose to "focus participants on shared examples and to increase the likelihood that divergent perceptions were likely to be real and not secondary to artifact" (p. 929). The rigor of designing a study and reporting its details, such as in the study by Musselman et al., ensures that information generated from study participants have validity.

How Are Research Data Analyzed?

The authors report that three reviewers analyzed the transcribed content including a surgical resident, an OR nurse, and a qualitative researcher. As a team, these reviewers read transcripts multiple times in an iterative and recursive manner, which is key to drawing out recurring themes that are present in transcripts. The full report of the article describes that reviewers initially identified high-level thematic categories, individually reviewed transcripts using the categories as a lens to organize the content, met on a regular basis to resolve disagreements, and finalized the coding categories including identifying specific examples and types of languages from the transcripts. As you can see, qualitative research largely depends on two factors during the content analysis process: (1) reviewers share a common understanding of research goals and (2) saturation of thematic codes is achieved by fully exploring meanings and relationship of information collected from subjects. This rigorous research process is critical to ensuring reliability of data reported in qualitative studies. As a complement to the content analysis process, Musselman et al. also reported that they used the NVivo qualitative software program for further examining interrelationships among thematic categories. It is important to remember that this type of software program does not create thematic categories for you. It simply takes the transcript materials and the categories researchers agree upon and helps facilitate more in-depth analyses of relationship among the categories.

How Are Research Data Reported?

Musselman et al. report their results in a descriptive manner around the themes of how surgeons and residents rationalize the positive impact of intimidation and harassment. This descriptive reporting of themes is accompanied with direct quotes from study participants to provide a context to the thematic meanings. The authors also provide a diagram (p. 931) that illustrates the interrelationship of themes in a conceptual framework that the authors labeled as *the legitimacy assessment model of rationalization*. If you are fairly new to qualitative research design, the study by Musselman et al. is an excellent example that demonstrates many levels of research rigor that are incorporated in both the study design and reporting.

Conclusion

In this chapter, we reviewed both quantitative and qualitative methodologies available to study various educational issues pertaining to training of students, residents, and practicing surgeons. The key messages of this chapter include the following: rigorous research rests on formulating a clear research goal, providing a justification for the number of subjects recruited in the study, pilot testing assessment instruments you are using for collecting data, reporting reliability and validity of scores collected from these instruments, and selecting the appropriate analytical methods for examining and analyzing your findings. At a time when a new learning emphasis is placed on nontechnical skills such as communication, professionalism, and leadership, the application of rigorous research methodologies we have described is of utmost importance to advance the science of education, thereby expanding our collective knowledge base of surgical educational practices.

References

1. Downing SM. Validity: on meaningful interpretation of assessment data. Med Educ. 2003;37(9):830–7.
2. Immenroth M, Bürger T, Brenner J, Nagelschmidt M, Eberspächer H, Troidl H. Mental training in surgical education: a randomized controlled trial. Ann Surg. 2007;245(3):385–91.
3. Musselman LJ, MacRae HM, Reznick RK, Lingard LA. 'You learn better under the gun': intimidation and harassment in surgical education. Med Educ. 2005;39(9):926–34.

Further Reading

Brennan RL. Generalizability theory. New York: Springer; 2001.

Kachigan SK. Multivariate statistical analyses. New York: Radius Press; 1991.

Krueger RA. Focus groups: a practical guide for applied research. Thousand Oaks: Sage Publications; 1994.

Martin P, Bateason P. Measuring behavior: an introductory guide. Cambridge: Cambridge University Press; 1993.

Martin JA, Regehr G, Reznick R, MacRae H, Murnaghan J, Hutchison C, Brown M. Objective structured assessment of technical skill (OSATS) for surgical residents. Br J Surg. 1997;84(2):273–8.

Merriam SB. Qualitative research and case study applications in education. Revised and expanded from "case study research in education". San Francisco: Jossey-Bass Publishers; 1998.

Murphy KR, Myors B, Wolach A. Statistical power analysis: a simple and general model for traditional and modern hypothesis tests. New York: Routledge/Academic; 2008.

Van Nortwick SS, Lendvay TS, Jensen AR, Wright AS, Horvath KD, Kim S. Methodologies for establishing validity in surgical simulation studies. Surgery. 2010;147(5):622–30.

Chapter 14
Research Funding

Dimitrios Stefanidis

Current Status of Medical Education Research

The continuous introduction of new techniques and procedures that must be mastered within the constraints of limited work hours and the rapid proliferation of medical knowledge has created the need for changes in surgical training. As a result, surgical education has seen a paradigm shift in recent years with emphasis being placed on training outside the operating room and identification of the most effective educational methods. These changes have also fueled a tremendous growth in medical education research as is evident by an increasing number of related publications. A systematic review of the literature on undergraduate medical education research found a tremendous increase in the number of publications from 1 during the 1969–1970 period to 147 during 2006–2007. Furthermore, it demonstrated an increasing methodological rigor of the published studies and also identified considerable opportunities for improvement. Similarly, studies assessing the surgical education literature have also demonstrated trends of increasing publication numbers and improved methodological rigor in addition to an increasing popularity of publications in peer-reviewed surgical journals (as opposed to educational journals).

Despite this documented growth in medical and surgical education research productivity, the funds dedicated to educational research are severely limited and may negatively impact this trend and the quality of published studies. Data from 1994

D. Stefanidis, MD, PhD, FACS
Department of Surgery, Carolinas Simulation Center,
Carolinas Healthcare System,
1025 Morehead Medical Dr, Suite 300,
Charlotte, NC 28204, USA
e-mail: dimitrios.stefanidis@carolinas.org

C.M. Pugh, R.S. Sippel (eds.), *Success in Academic Surgery:*
Developing a Career in Surgical Education, Success in Academic Surgery,
DOI 10.1007/978-1-4471-4691-9_14, © Springer-Verlag London 2013

and 1998 show that less than 0.001–0.01 % of federal spending in graduate medical education was used for educational research. Furthermore, a more recent survey of first authors of medical education studies published during 2002–2003 demonstrated that the majority of published research was not formally funded and the studies that received support were substantially underfunded (30 % of studies had received funding that was, on average, less than half their actual cost). Factors independently associated with attaining funding included training in grant writing and number of medical education studies published by the first author. Importantly, the same authors found that smaller amounts of grant funding were associated with inferior quality of medical education research.

The objective of this chapter is to provide information on available funding sources for medical education research and offer readers with suggestions for successful funding.

Funding Sources

In general, most of the funding for surgical and medical research comes from industry and the federal government. Additionally, national professional organizations, charitable organizations, and state and institutional sources may also fund research. The majority of funding sources seek out specific proposals of interest to them. Funding for unsolicited proposals, while possible, tends to be scarce. While limited, funding for educational research may be obtained from a variety of well sought-out sources for appropriate proposals. Investigators should initially examine local resources, as many institutions offer small amounts of funding for pilot research projects that can be also used for medical education research. Such funding is intended for the generation of preliminary data that will support applications for funding by external sources. Asking more experienced research colleagues for input, seeking out the funding sources of published educational research studies, and searching the Internet can also help identify existing funding opportunities for projects of interest to the educational researcher. In addition, a number of national medical specialty societies offer competitive grants for education research, but the awards are generally modest. Even though government funding for educational research is sporadic, the federal government is still the major source of funds for medical education development and research, through a variety of training programs across a number of agencies. Training grants, career awards, fellowships, and scholarships are available from many federal agencies. While many of these grants do not fund medical education research per se, they may provide opportunities to develop and evaluate educational programs as well as to learn and develop skills in research methods. Industry supports the majority of research in the USA and can, on occasion, also provide funding for education research projects.

The following is a list of available funding sources in the USA for educational research. Hyperlinks are provided for easy access to more detailed information. The reader is advised to access the individual funding agency websites as the information provided here may become outdated over time. Special reference is made to search engines for research funding in medicine.

Online Search Engines for Grant Funding (None Specific to Medical Education)

Community of Science (COS): http://www.cos.com/

This is the most comprehensive source of funding information available on the Web, with more than 23,000 records representing over 400,000 funding opportunities totaling over $33 billion.

Grants.gov: http://www.grants.gov/

Grants.gov is the single access point for over 900 grant programs offered by the 26 federal grant-making agencies.

GrantsNet: http://www.hhs.gov/grantsnet/

This Web-based application tool provides information on 300 Department of Health and Human Services (HHS) and other federal grant programs.

The Foundation Center: http://foundationcenter.org/

The Foundation Center seeks to advance knowledge about US philanthropy. The center conducts and facilitates research on trends in the field and maintains a database on more than 2.3 million grants and more than 75,000 currently active grant makers.

ResearchResearch: http://www.researchresearch.com/

This site provides news and information for the international research community. It offers in-depth news coverage of research policy and politics and comprehensive listings of funding opportunities and sponsors across all disciplines.

Funding Sources Specific to Surgical Education

A few surgical societies offer grants that can be used for educational research projects.

CESERT Grant: Association for Surgical Education

The best example is the Center for Excellence in Surgical Education, Research and Training (CESERT) grant offered by the Association for Surgical Education Foundation. These grants aim to disseminate funds that support innovative research and education projects and programs, which will advance surgical education in North America. Association for Surgical Education (ASE) members are given funding priority, but non-ASE members can also apply in collaboration with an ASE member.

Funding priorities include Innovations in Surgical Education that Improve Patient Care Research, Innovations in Performance Evaluation and Assessment, Innovations in Medical Student Programs, Innovations in Resident and Faculty Development, and Innovations in Educational Administration.

The level of funding is currently up to $25,000 for the duration of the project. Submission deadline is on June 1st.

Detailed information can be obtained at http://www.surgicaleducation.com/cesert-grants

Roslyn Faculty Research Award: Association of Academic Surgeons

The intent of this award is to provide early-career research support to junior faculty members of the AAS. It is awarded every other year. Applicants must be full-time faculty who are within 5 years of completion of their surgical training, have not yet attained the rank of Associate Professor, and have a mentor who is AAS member. These grants are not specific to educational research but such projects might be considered. The level of funding is $35,000 for 1 year to be used for direct cost expenditures incurred in the conduct of the proposed research project but not for salary support. Deadline is typically in early September.

Detailed information can be obtained at http://www.aasurg.org/awards/award_roslyn.php

AAS Research Fellowship Award

The intent of these awards is to provide an eligible resident or fellow who is engaged in clinical outcomes, health services, or education research the opportunity to spend 1 year in a full-time basic research position with an AAS member. Applicants must have completed at least 2 years of postgraduate training in a surgical discipline. The award of $20,000 for 1 year may be used for salary support or for the direct cost expenditures of the research. Submission deadline is typically in early September.

Detailed information can be obtained at http://www.aasurg.org/awards/fellowship_award_research.php

Society of University Surgeons (SUS) Resident Scholar Award

The SUS Resident Scholar Award is a 1 year $30,000 research grant intended for surgical residents in any of the surgical disciplines who are doing research focused on surgical innovation, bioengineering, or surgical education utilizing new technologies. The application deadline is usually in April.

Detailed information can be obtained at http://www.susweb.org/sus-resident-scholar-award

The SUS Junior Faculty Award

This $30,000 research grant is sponsored annually by the SUS Foundation for 1 year with the possibility to extend it another year. It targets surgical faculty members who are within their first 3 years of appointment in a tenure track faculty position following postgraduate training and is intended to support the research of a surgeon whose work involves the basic science that underlies a surgical disease. Whether educational research projects are acceptable is unclear. Submission deadline is usually in August.

Detailed information can be obtained at http://www.susweb.org/junior-faculty-award

SAGES Research Grants and Career Development Awards

Another society that often awards grants for education research is the Society of American Gastrointestinal and Endoscopic Surgeons (SAGES). The funding level is up to $30,000. These grants focus on stimulating original research in gastrointestinal and endoscopic surgery. In general, the topics chosen for funding are based on a research agenda that was developed by the SAGES membership. Two of the top 20 identified research questions related to education research include: "What methods of simulation are most effective in helping surgeons learn techniques and skills for gastrointestinal and endoscopic surgery?" and "What are the best objective methods for measuring surgical proficiency?" The deadline for grant submission is in November. SAGES also offers a career development award in the amount of $60,000 that could be applied to continued education in educational research methods.

Detailed information can be obtained at http://sages.org/leadership/committees/research/grants.php

American College of Surgeons (ACS) Resident Research Scholarship

The American College of Surgeons is offering 2-year resident research scholarships. Eligibility for these scholarships is limited to the research projects of residents in surgery or a surgical specialty. The applicant must be a resident member of the college who has completed two postdoctoral years in an accredited surgical training program in the United States or Canada at the time the scholarship is awarded and shall not complete formal residency training before completion of the award. The scholarship is $30,000 per year and is to support the research but not salary. Application deadline is in early September.

Detailed information can be obtained at http://www.facs.org/memberservices/acsresident.html

American College of Surgeons Faculty Research Fellowship

The American College of Surgeons is offering 2-year faculty research fellowships to surgeons entering academic careers in surgery or a surgical specialty. The fellowship is to assist a surgeon in the establishment of a new and independent research program. Applicants should have demonstrated their potential to work as independent investigators. The fellowship award is $40,000 per year for each of 2 years to support the research but not the salary of the applicant. Preference is given to applicants who directly enter academic surgery following residency or fellowship. Application deadline is in November.

Detailed information can be obtained at http://www.facs.org/memberservices/acsfaculty.html

Other Educational Research Funding Sources

AERA Grants Program

The American Educational Research Association (AERA) with support from the National Science Foundation (NSF) awards grants of $20,000–$35,000 to education researchers whose projects are quantitative in nature; include the analysis of existing data from NCES, NSF, or other federal agencies; and have US education policy relevance. The program also offers training to researchers through its annual training institutes. There are three funding cycles.

Detailed   information   can   be   obtained   at   http://www.aera.net/ProfessionalOpportunitiesFunding/FundingOpportunities/AERAGrantsProgram/ResearchGrants/tabid/12813/Default.aspx

Agency for Healthcare Research and Quality

The Agency for Healthcare Research and Quality (AHRQ) supports a broad program of health services research and works with partners to promote improvements in clinical and health systems practices that benefit patients. Along these lines, some education research projects may be funded. In 2006 and 2010, the agency issued requests for applications (RFAs) for research aimed to improve patient safety using simulation. Besides simulation, other education research requests specific to areas of interest to the agency may be issued. A list of previously funded projects is available on the AHRQ Web site via a searchable database that is named GOLD (Grants On-Line Database).

Detailed information can be obtained at http://www.ahrq.gov/fund/

Stemmler Medical Education Research Fund

This fund is offered by the National Board of Medical Examiners (NBME) and supports research or development of innovative assessment approaches that enhance the evaluation of persons preparing to or continuing to practice medicine. Funding is made available to both pilot and more comprehensive projects. Requests for up to $150,000 for a project period of up to 2 years are considered. Submission deadline is typically in May for letters of intent and July for full proposals if requested.

Detailed information can be obtained at http://www.nbme.org/research/stemmler.html

Philip Manning Research Grant in Continuing Medical Education

The Research Endowment Council of the Society for Academic Continuing Medical Education (SACME) sponsors original research studies related to physician lifelong learning and physician change. Submitted proposals must use either quantitative or qualitative methods in a rigorous scientific design. One award of up to $50,000 is made every 2 years for proposals lasting 2 years. Initially a letter of intent must be submitted and be accompanied by a letter of support from the director of the CME program at a SACME member's organization.

Detailed information can be obtained at http://www.sacme.org/SACME_grants

Fund for the Improvement of Post-secondary Education

The Institute of Education Sciences of the US Department of Education offers funding opportunities for education research that contributes to improved academic achievement for all students, and particularly for minorities. The institute supports a series of specific research programs and also accepts unsolicited research applications. A little more interesting and relevant to medical education may be the annual competition for the "Fund for the Improvement of Postsecondary Education (FIPSE)" grant that is designed to support innovative reform projects that hold promise as models for the resolution of important issues and problems in postsecondary education. These grants may be in support of any academic discipline, program, or student support service.

Detailed information can be obtained at http://www.ed.gov/programs/fipsecomp/index.html

Southern Group on Educational Affairs

The Southern Group on Educational Affairs (SGEA) of the Association of American Medical Colleges (AAMC) supports and encourages scholarship in medical education by sponsoring small educational research projects. The SGEA provides up to two $3,000 research grants per year to be used to create new opportunities for its members to initiate research projects. Submission deadline is typically in July.

Detailed information can be obtained at https://www.aamc.org/members/gea/regions/sgea/awards/66884/sgea_research.html

AACOM Medical Education Mini-research Grants

The American Association of Colleges of Osteopathic Medicine (AACOM) supports small medical education research grants. Applicants must be educators at Colleges of Osteopathic Medicine, including their OPTI programs. Proposals are supported to the maximum amount of $10,000 for 1 year, and the submission deadline is in early January.

Detailed information can be obtained at http://www.aacom.org/InfoFor/educators/Pages/aacomgrants.aspx

Other Potential Funding Sources

National Institute of Health: http://grants.nih.gov/grants/guide/index.html

Although the NIH does not have a specified funding category for education research, appropriate projects may be funded if they fall under any of its supported research programs. One example that targets mainly K-12 education is the NIH NCRR Science Education Partnership Award (SEPA) (R25):

http://grants.nih.gov/grants/guide/pa-files/PAR-10-206.html

Health Resources and Services Administration: http://www.hrsa.gov/grants/default.htm

The Health Resources and Services Administration (HRSA) of the Department of Health and Human Services offers funding for health professions education and training programs. The agency makes funds available to support Area Health Education Centers. Education research projects may be funded under some of its programs.

National Science Foundation: http://www.nsf.gov/dir/index.jsp?org=ehr

The National Science Foundation (NSF) accounts for about 20 % of federal support for basic research conducted by America's colleges and universities. Under its education and research program, the foundation may fund education research projects.

The Josiah Macy Jr. Foundation: http://www.josiahmacyfoundation.org/

The Josiah Macy Jr. Foundation supports programs designed to improve the education of health professionals in the interest of the health of the public and to enhance the representation of minorities in the health profession. Funding priorities include:

(1) projects to improve medical and health professional education in the context of the changing healthcare system, (2) projects that will increase diversity among healthcare professionals, (3) projects that demonstrate or encourage ways to increase teamwork among healthcare professionals, and (4) educational strategies to increase care for underserved populations. The foundation requires a three-page preliminary letter of inquiry that includes a description of the project, the names and qualifications of the responsible individuals, and an initial budget before submission of a full proposal. Grants are made to tax-exempt institutions or agencies only and not directly to individuals. There is no specified deadline for proposal submission.

W. K. Kellogg Foundation: http://www.wkkf.org/

The mission of the W. K. Kellogg Foundation is to create communities, systems, and nations in which all children have an equitable and promising future and can thrive. The foundation provides grants to tax-exempt organizations but not to individuals. One of its priorities is education and learning.

Other funding agencies that might support educational research projects include:

Rockefeller Foundation: http://www.rockfound.org/grants/grants.shtml
Robert Wood Johnson Foundation: http://www.rwjf.org/grants/
Henry J. Kaiser Family Foundation: http://www.kff.org/
PEW Charitable Trust: http://www.pewtrusts.org/program_investments.aspx
Arnold P. Gold Foundation: http://humanism-in-medicine.org/index.php/programs_grants
Arthur Vining Davis Foundation: http://www.avdf.org/FoundationsPrograms/HealthCare.aspx
George Washington Institute for Spirituality & Health (Gwish): http://www.gwumc.edu/gwish/awards/index.cfm

Industry-Sponsored Grants

Some industry partners may also provide grant funding for education research-related projects. Several examples include the AstraZeneca, Genentech, and Pfizer medical education grants, which sponsor projects related to patient education and also projects that examine the effectiveness of such educational efforts.

Detailed information can be obtained at

http://www.astrazenecagrants.com/
http://www.gene.com/gene/imed/areas-interest.html
http://www.pfizer.com/responsibility/grants_contributions/medical_education_grants.jsp

Strategies for Successful Funding

The first step for a successful project is the identification of an important problem or need and the related research question that could solve the problem or cover the need. Personal experience, exchange of ideas with colleagues, or a review of the relevant medical education literature will usually provide a list of problems and needs that lend themselves for further research. The next step is to identify the funding source and start planning the application process. A diligent search for the most appropriate funding agency with an interest in the applicant's project and careful review of its submission requirements and of prior funded projects will make it clear if it is appropriate for the project. Alternatively, if a funding source is already known or a call for proposals has been issued, review of the objectives and areas of interest of the funding agency will provide an excellent starting point for the formulation of research questions. Assessing the feasibility of the conceived project should occur at this point at the latest; a careful assessment of personal strengths and weaknesses, available institutional resources and support, potential collaborations that could enhance the project, and time commitment required will clarify the feasibility of the project. It is very important that the applicant is realistic about the time and effort required to prepare the application and to complete the project. In general, it takes about 1 year to collect preliminary data, 1–2 months for Institutional Review Board and/or Institutional Animal Care and Use Committee approval, 1–2 months to write the grant, 5–6 months from submission to review, 1–2 months to receive the review and decision, and about 9 months from grant submission to funding.

When the decision has been made to submit an application to the appropriate funding agency, the applicant should strictly observe the application format and requirements and submission timeline. While the format may vary from agency to agency, a grant proposal should generally include an abstract/project summary, background and significance, preliminary work, hypothesis and specific aims, research design and methods, budget, assurances, available resources, and investigator curriculum vitae. Applicants should clearly demonstrate in their proposal what they want to accomplish, the steps they will take, the methods they will use, and the measures of project success. Moreover, applicants should demonstrate their maturity as researchers by identifying potential research problems or barriers that may be encountered and propose ways to prevent or overcome them when they occur. Applicants should highlight the scientific merit of their proposal and convince reviewers that their study is absolutely necessary for the common good, has strong potential to lead to further studies or funding, and that they are the ideal team to take on this project. An important strategy is to seek collaboration and outside expertise to compensate for potential weaknesses of the primary investigators and assemble a team to help with the application process (researchers, writers, proofreaders). Seeking advice, help, and criticism from seasoned grant writers will improve the proposal and increase its chance for acceptance. Perhaps the most important ingredient for success, however, is being persistent; if a proposal is rejected, carefully analyze the reviewers' comments, address fixable problems, and resubmit a revised stronger proposal to the same or a different agency. It takes time and dedication to get projects funded and, often, the road to success is paved with failures.

On the other hand, if the grant is awarded, the project must be implemented in a timely manner and the money accounted for and spent properly. Execution of the proposal takes much time and effort, which the applicant should have already planned for.

Epilogue

While funding for medical education research is limited, a diligent search for funding sources such as the ones referenced in this chapter is likely to identify opportunities that meet the needs of the educational researcher. When the funding source has been identified, attention to the application requirements and timelines involved are extremely important for the submission of a successful application. Applicant persistence and determination are the most important virtues of the successful educational researcher.

Further Reading

Baernstein A, Liss HK, Carney PA, Elmore JG. Trends in study methods used in undergraduate medical education research, 1969–2007. JAMA. 2007;298:1038–45.

Carline JD. Funding medical education research: opportunities and issues. Acad Med. 2004;79:918–24.

Derossis AM, DaRosa DA, Dutta S, Dunnington GL. A ten-year analysis of surgical education research. Am J Surg. 2000;180:58–61.

Reed DA, Kern DE, Levine RB, Wright SM. Costs and funding for published medical education research. JAMA. 2005;294:1052–57.

Reed DA, Cook DA, Beckman TJ, Levine RB, Kern DE, Wright SM. Association between funding and quality of published medical education research. JAMA. 2007;298:1002–9.

Chapter 15
Getting Your Work Published

Melina C. Vassiliou, Liane S. Feldman, and Gerald M. Fried

Publishing the results of scholarly work is critical for the development of any academic career. In surgical education research, contributions to the peer-reviewed literature have increased significantly in the past decades, and this has helped "legitimize" education research as an academic focus [1]. In addition to the traditional avenues for publication of research endeavors, such as conference presentations and journals, other academic work in surgical education, including teaching and assessment materials, can be disseminated through Internet-based resources. This provides an important opportunity for career development for the surgical educator who may not have a research focus. In either case, submitting your work for publication requires you to formally organize the work and put it in the context of what was done before, anticipate comments and questions, and make it understandable to a wide audience, thereby developing as a researcher and educator. The ultimate goal is to allow others to learn from and build on your experiences, both positive and negative, while developing an academic portfolio that will objectively demonstrate your contributions in surgical education. In this chapter, we will first discuss publication of surgical education research in journals and through other traditional venues and then focus on the dissemination of other educational work, such as curricula and assessments, through less traditional forms of publication.

M.C. Vassiliou, MD, MED (✉) • L.S. Feldman, MD • G.M. Fried, MD
Department of Surgery, Division of General Surgery,
McGill University Health Centre,
Montreal, QC, Canada
e-mail: melina.vassiliou@mcgill.ca

C.M. Pugh, R.S. Sippel (eds.), *Success in Academic Surgery:* 137
Developing a Career in Surgical Education, Success in Academic Surgery,
DOI 10.1007/978-1-4471-4691-9_15, © Springer-Verlag London 2013

Conference-Based Publications

Presentation of academic work at surgical or education conferences is a very effective strategy for publication. This has been the most common approach to publication in our careers. There are several roads to publication related to conferences. As with other research endeavors, the most common strategy is submission of an abstract in advance of the meeting. An abstract is a synopsis of the research project and findings. The peer-review process for the abstract can give the young researcher important feedback for the work. Presentation at the conference has the added value of enabling networking with other researchers in your field and gaining exposure for yourself and your work. Many societies will have an expedited review process with a specific journal to facilitate publication of work presented at the conference. This information should be reviewed at the time of abstract submission. In some cases, it is a requirement to submit the manuscript to that journal when the abstract is selected for presentation at the conference. The journal will complete a second, full peer-review process to decide on publication, but often this is expedited as an accepted abstract has already gone through peer review when presented at the meeting.

In this conference-based strategy, the opportunity to present your research to a wide audience is based on a summary of your work, rather than the entire manuscript. This can have advantages early on in a research program. It is important that the abstract be an effective summary of your project. The format is specified by the society and must be followed. An interesting title will attract the reviewer's interest. The introduction should highlight the importance of the research question in one or two sentences. Methods should be as succinct as possible so that the emphasis of the abstract is the results. A figure or small table can be an effective way to summarize data. The conclusion must follow from the data and should focus on the practical applications of the results. Spelling errors, failure to define units, jargon, excessive reference to your previous work, conclusions not supported by the results, and promises of work to come detract from the abstract and reduce the likelihood of acceptance [2].

Each coauthor should review the abstract. We find it useful to read the abstract in a meeting with as many coauthors present as possible. One cannot be too thin skinned; the revision process makes the abstract better. Ask experienced colleagues and researchers to review the abstract, even if they do not have a specific interest in surgical education. It may be useful to have the opinion of your division chief or department chair, as this both provides feedback and allows them to understand your work and productivity level. Duplicate submissions, where the same abstract or significantly overlapping abstracts are submitted to more than one venue simultaneously, is a serious ethical violation.

It is important to know the focus of the society to which the work is submitted to direct the work appropriately and to present the findings in a way that makes them relevant to the readership. Even the best quality abstract will not be accepted if the work is not aligned or is inconsistent with the interests and values of the sponsoring society. Attending meetings is a good way to understand the interests of the

Table 15.1 Surgical meetings with a focus on education or sections devoted to education

Organization/meeting	Focus	Official journal
Association for Surgical Education (ASE)	Surgical education	American Journal of Surgery
Association of Program Directors in Surgery (APDS)	Postgraduate surgical education	Journal of Surgical Education
Association for Academic Surgery (AAS)	Research-based academic surgery	Journal of Surgical Research
Society of University Surgeons (SUS)	Research-based academic surgery	Surgery
American College of Surgeons – Surgical Forum (ACS)	Research, including education section	Journal of the American College of Surgeons
American College of Surgeons – Accredited Education Institutes – Annual Consortium Meeting	Surgical simulation	Surgery
Society of American Gastrointestinal and Endoscopic Surgeons (SAGES)	Minimally invasive surgery	Surgical Endoscopy
International Conference on Surgical Education and Training (ICOSET)	Postgraduate surgical education	
World Congress on Surgical Training http://www.surgicon.org/	International, postgraduate, and CME	

sponsoring society. Reviewing meeting programs, abstract books, and journal manuscripts from recent meetings, available at the society's website, can help identify topics and methodologies of interest. One needs to understand the type of work that has been presented at the meeting in recent years. A mentor can be very valuable in helping to identify appropriate venues for the work. There are several surgical societies with a particular interest in education, and many other clinical societies will devote a segment of the meeting to education. Some examples from our experience are listed in Table 15.1. In addition, there are general medical education and simulation meetings that may be interested in your work and that may provide opportunities to collaborate across disciplines. For example, many simulation meetings attract other health professionals, engineers, kinesiologists, educational psychologists, psychometricians, and information technology specialists to name a few. Some of these meetings are listed in Table 15.2; however, this list is certainly not exhaustive.

Presenting at society meetings is an opportunity to meet other investigators in your field. Meetings generally cluster related topics in specific sessions. Whether at the podium or at a poster presentation, people attending the session are interested in your work. This allows you to present to your peers, address questions, and build a reputation. The opportunity to ask respectful and insightful questions of other investigators also helps gain exposure. The chair of the session is usually a recognized leader in the field, and offline discussions may follow from these sessions and create opportunities for collaboration. This can be especially helpful if one does not have those opportunities or mentorship at home.

Video presentations are welcome at some meetings. Traditionally these have focused on specific surgical techniques with limited academic value. However,

Table 15.2 Medical education and simulation meetings

Organization	Meeting	Focus	Journal/publication
An International Association for Medical Education – AMEE	Ottawa Conference	Best evidence guidelines, cross-discipline collaboration	*Medical Teacher*, *MedEdWorld* (online), *MedEdCentral* (online)
		Assessment of competence	*Medical Teacher*
Association of American Medical Colleges https://www.aamc.org/	Annual meeting and others	Continuing medical education and education research	*Academic Medicine*
Royal College of Physicians and Surgeons of Canada	International Conference on Residency Education	Postgraduate	
	Simulation Summit	Simulation	
Society for Simulation in Healthcare	International Meeting on Simulation in Healthcare (IMSH)	Simulation education, assessment, and integration	*Simulation in Healthcare*
MedBiquitous	Annual meeting	Technology standards for healthcare education and competence assessment	
American College of Surgeons	Annual Meeting of the Accredited Education Institutes	Simulation, surgical training and assessment	*Surgery*
NextMed	Medicine Meets Virtual Reality (MMVR)	Advanced medical technologies, Simulation	*Studies in Health Technology and Informatics*

grounding technical videos in educational theory can enhance their value. Videos that showcase innovative educational approaches, such as the setup of a novel simulation or curriculum, also have significant potential to showcase your work in action. In the context of a meeting, videos are peer reviewed and the abstract published, which contributes to an academic portfolio.

In addition to abstract submission, involvement in surgical or education societies can lead to publications through other mechanisms. All surgical societies will have one or more education committees, charged with CME, resident education, training, assessment, or special projects. Involvement on an education committee provides opportunities to create and publish guidelines, surveys, position statements, or books/manuals representing the work of the committee. Some committees may be charged with creating educational material (e.g., SAGES "Fundamentals" committees, including Fundamentals of Laparoscopic Surgery (FLS)), which then provide access to multicenter collaborations and data related to the project. Volunteering for projects (and delivering results) is an excellent way to enhance one's national and international reputation and create other opportunities to showcase one's work.

Proposing and planning a workshop at an education conference is another avenue for publication. Workshops are featured prominently at the Association of Program Directors in Surgery (APDS) and the Royal College of Physicians and Surgeons of Canada Simulation Summit and International Conference on Surgical Education and Training. The content of the workshop can then be collated and submitted for publication, usually in the journal associated with the sponsoring society.

Nonconference-Based Publications

It is important to select an appropriate journal for submission of your research manuscript. One begins thinking about where the work will be submitted when designing the study. The manuscript should then be written following the format for the chosen journal. The goal is to publish in the "best" journal possible for the quality of the research in order to have the widest impact. Not every journal publishes research in surgical education. Several categories of journals can be identified that might publish surgical education research: general medical journals, general surgical journals, specialty-specific surgical journals, medical education journals, and journals dedicated to surgical education or with a specific focus in surgical education. Most research in surgical education is published in surgery journals as opposed to general medical education journals [1].

Selection of a specific journal for submission will depend on the scope of the journal and the quality of the research. Success at a general surgical or medical journal requires research questions and results of sufficiently broad interest. The best way to begin to get a sense of the scope of a journal is to scan the table of contents regularly. This provides information on whether surgical education research is published by the journal, whether there is a focus on education, what level of education is discussed (i.e., undergraduate, postgraduate, CME), and what types of research methodologies are used (i.e., qualitative versus quantitative). The quality of the work and whether it will fit with the journal's audience can be judged by seeking advice from a mentor or senior collaborator.

Articles published in open-access journals are available online to anyone, usually without financial barriers. Some are subsidized, while others require payment from authors. There are advantages and disadvantages to these journals. The upside is that the research presented is accessible to everyone and can increase readership and citations. The downside is the potential threat to the integrity of the peer-review process. A directory of open-access journals can be found at http://www.doaj.org/.

The acceptance of a paper after peer review is always a thrill and brings a sense of pride and accomplishment related to the fact that someone else sees the value and relevance of your work. On the other hand, the rejection of a manuscript always stings. Instead of simply resubmitting to a lower-impact journal, put the rejected manuscript aside for a few days and then come back to it when the hurt has subsided. The reviewers' comments and reasons for the rejection can almost always be used in a constructive way to improve the quality of the work. After revisions and improvements, it may be accepted by a journal of similar quality to the one that originally declined publication.

Another opportunity is to do a well-researched structured review of a topic in surgical education. These reviews are excellent learning opportunities and, when well done, provide great value to the reader by organizing available data and evaluating the quality of the information. Such reviews provide ideas for further research and position the author as an expert on the topic.

An excellent way to understand the process of selection for journals in your field is to become a journal reviewer. Opportunities to review work may arise from senior colleagues and mentors, from involvement in specialty societies, through the process of submission of manuscripts to a journal, or from being suggested as a reviewer by another researcher. Reviewing manuscripts takes a lot of time but helps develop expertise, critical thinking, and an understanding of selection criteria. It is also an important academic contribution and is the cornerstone of the peer-review process.

Other Publication Opportunities

In addition to submitting abstracts and manuscripts, one may be invited to contribute to a body of work. Examples include textbook chapters, papers for special journal issues, or manuscripts arising from invited talks at conferences. Early on in one's career, these opportunities usually arise through a mentor recommending you or asking for your collaboration. These are generally not peer reviewed but have a prestige factor related to the widespread use of the textbook or from being in the company of other well-known contributors. There are many demands on your time, but contributing within your field of research is time well spent. Involvement at the committee level in specialty organizations also may lead to opportunities to moderate conference sessions or panels. As chair, one may then ask the other panelists to contribute manuscripts of their talks that can be collated into a special paper that can be submitted to the specialty's journal.

Publishing Work Other than Surgical Education Research

Surgical education is an increasingly popular field and involves creation of and participation in many scholarly projects that may not take the form of traditional academic research. Examples include courses, curricula, assessment instruments, teaching resources, uses of educational technologies, instructional strategies, and simulators or simulation scenarios. In addition, innovative solutions to some current education problems in surgery such as work-hour restrictions, new training requirements, or continuing medical education challenges may also be an area in which you have some expertise. Getting this work published and recognized is important for career advancement and as a way for others to benefit and learn from it. Sometimes, with some minor modifications, many of these items can be converted into small research or pilot projects that could be appropriate for publication in peer-reviewed journals. The addition of an assessment or user questionnaire to a curriculum or the validation of a new assessment instrument would be some common examples. In addition, several journals will publish case studies or reports describing a new education program, simulator, or application of an educational theory or framework to some aspect of surgical education. Editorials can also be a way to introduce a new idea or perspective on a surgical education topic, but selection of the appropriate journal and audience is key. Furthermore, if you are pursuing an education degree or taking a course, some of the efforts you put into completing a course, such as a final paper, review, or essay, can be published. Some examples of print and online journals that consider these types of scholarly work are included in Table 15.3. Please consult the individual websites of each journal for the criteria and rules of submission.

Less Traditional Ways of Getting Your Work Published

Several societies and organizations have started to recognize the importance of scholarly education contributions and provide opportunities for sharing and online publication. The most widely known among these is MedEdPORTAL https://www.mededportal.org/. MedEdPORTAL is a free online, peer-reviewed publication service offered by the Association of American Medical Colleges. The goal is to provide a forum for exchange of educational resources and collaboration among healthcare professionals. Education videos, curricula, assessments, essays, and other medical education-related content can be submitted. They maintain a rigorous

Table 15.3 Selected journals that may consider scholarly education work in forms other than original research

Journal of Surgical Education
Surgical Innovation
Simulation in Healthcare
Medical Teacher
Medical Education
Teaching and Learning in Medicine
Life Sciences Education (online) http://www.lifescied.org/site/misc/ifora.xhtml
Bioscience Education (online) http://www.bioscience.heacademy.ac.uk/journal/

peer-review process but are not currently indexed in PubMed. This may change in the near future and is a goal they are working towards. MedEdPORTAL also allows users to download a usage report, which can be used for academic promotion purposes. It lists who downloaded your resource and what they intended to use it for. MedEdPORTAL, in partnership with the Georgia Health Sciences University, is also creating a Directory and Repository of Educational Assessment Measures (*DREAM*), a peer-reviewed searchable database of health education assessment tools. They plan to launch DREAM in 2013. Information about the submission process for those interested in contributing is available at https://www.mededportal.org/about/initiatives/dream/developer/.

In addition to MedEdPORTAL, there are several other web-based surgical education initiatives that may be interested in your work. WISE-MD – the Web Initiative for Surgical Education – was initially designed to address gaps in medical student education related to the shift towards outpatient care. It harnesses the educational power of animations, videos, and other technologies to enhance learning. If you would like to contribute a module to this resource, consider contacting the leadership of WISE-MD http://wise-md.med.nyu.edu/wmd_leader.jsp. Some other online surgical education resources are listed in Table 15.4.

Even Less Traditional Ways of Sharing and Publicizing Your Ideas

There are myriad novel ways to publish and share your ideas and work as a surgical educator. The concept of publication is undergoing a radical shift with the ubiquitous availability of opportunities to make one's work public and available on the web. These less traditional methods are currently not officially recognized by most

Table 15.4 Selected online surgical education resources

Online surgical education resource	Comments
SAGES University – through the SAGES Continuing Education Committee	A work-in-progress online resource to meet the CME needs of surgeons through journal clubs, online self-assessment programs, and other educational resources
SCORE – Surgical Council on Resident Education http://www.surgicalcore.org/index.html	Ongoing collaboration among several surgical societies to create a standard national curriculum. Includes a sophisticated learning management system. You might be able to contribute through one of the member societies
ACS/APDS Surgical Skills Curriculum for Residents http://www.facs.org/education/surgicalskills.html	Developed jointly by the American College of Surgeons and the Association of Program Directors in Surgery. Includes three phases: phase 1, basic surgical skills; phase 2, advanced skills and procedures; and phase 3, team-based skills

universities as scholarly work, but this may change with growing recognition of the value of Web 2.0 technologies as powerful media for communication and dissemination of information. Many enable contributors to track how many times their resource was accessed and what the potential impact might be. As per Wikipedia, "A Web 2.0 site allows users to interact and collaborate with each other in a social media dialogue as creators (prosumers) of user-generated content in a virtual community, in contrast to websites where users (consumers) are limited to the passive viewing of content that was created for them. Examples of Web 2.0 include social networking sites, blogs, wikis, video sharing sites, hosted services, web applications, mashups and folksonomies" (http://en.wikipedia.org/wiki/Web_2.0; accessed on September 3, 2012). The SAGES Surgical Wiki is one example of a Web 2.0 technology seeking contributions at http://www.sageswiki.org/. There are other surgical wikis springing up all over the web. The challenge for the host sites will be ensuring quality and accuracy, which, if one considers the Wikipedia model, is built into the design. Twitter is another Web 2.0 resource, also known as a microblog, that may be an interesting forum for surgical educators to share ideas, tricks, and tips that have worked for them. There are many examples of physician blogs and virtual communities that have been recognized as valuable educational resources and tools for students, residents, and colleagues all over the world. Patients, surgeons, and surgical trainees frequently refer to online videos and posts to learn about surgical procedures and diseases. If the content is of high quality, it is very likely to be found, used, and appreciated by the surgical community at large. It is evident that one must adhere to the highest ethical standards when contributing content to these websites and that patient confidentiality must be preserved and respected at all times. The opportunities to publish – in the unconventional use of the term – are unlimited, and the web is forever changing the way that we use, share, and evaluate information.

Conclusion

Surgical education is a fascinating, rich, and relatively young academic focus. It is becoming increasingly accepted as a research discipline, and the importance of the work in this field in improving the way we take care of patients is clear. People are interested in your work and want to hear about it, read about it, and discuss it with you. Presenting at meetings and participating in societies interested in surgical education is one of the most effective ways to promote your career and gain recognition in the field. Taking the time to craft an excellent abstract will go a long way. Select journals that are in alignment with your work, and use the reviewer comments to make your research better. Consider publishing other scholarly education work on MedEdPORTAL and other online collections of education resources. Finally, judicious use of Web 2.0 technologies may provide unprecedented and creative opportunities to collaborate and disseminate your work.

References

1. Dutta S, Dunnington GL. Factors contributing to success in surgical education research. Am J Surg. 2000;179:247–9.
2. Pruitt Jr BA, Mason Jr AD. Getting your abstract on the program. In: Troidl H, McKneally MF, Mulder DS, Troidl H, McKneally MF, Mulder DS, et al., editors. Surgical research: basic principles and clinical practice. 3rd ed. New York: Springer; 1998. p. 105–9.

Further Reading

Sanfey H, Gantt NL. Career development resource: academic career in surgical education. Am J Surg. 2012;204:126–9.

Index

C.M. Pugh, R.S. Sippel (eds.), *Success in Academic Surgery:*
Developing a Career in Surgical Education, Success in Academic Surgery,
DOI 10.1007/978-1-4471-4691-9, © Springer-Verlag London 2013

Printed by Printforce, the Netherlands